Surviving Natural Disasters
and Man-Made Disasters

Surviving Natural Disasters and Man-Made Disasters

Janice McCann and Betsy Shand

Resolution Press
Portland, Oregon

Resolution Press
8301 SW 6th Avenue
Portland, OR 97219
www.naturaldisastersbook.com

Copyright 2011 by Janice McCann and Betsy Shand

All rights reserved. Published 2011.
No part of this book may be used or reproduced in any manner whatsoever without written permission from the publisher. Neither the authors nor publisher assumes any responsibility for the use or misuse of information contained in this book. The authors have made every effort to provide accurate Internet addresses at the time of publication. The authors and publisher do not have any control over and do not assume any responsibility for third-party websites or their content or use.

For information on quantity discounts to corporations, schools, associations and groups, please contact publisher.

Printed in the United States of America

ISBN print book: 978-0-9838886-0-4
ISBN e-book: 978-0-9838886-1-1
Library of Congress Control Number: 2011936893

Editor: Heather Strang
Cover design: Bruce DeRoos
Interior design: Jennifer Omner
Website design: Russell Mickler, CISSP, Principal, Mickler and Associates, Inc.; and Bret Van Horn, The Workshed, Camas, WA.

Dedication

We dedicate this book to our inspirational and civic-minded mothers, Barbara Whipple McCann and Mary Anne Shand. They led us on the path to helping others by setting shining examples of duty, service, and volunteerism. Their involvement spanned college public service radio, Chamber of Commerce merchant to community outreach, coordination of Heart Association volunteers, leading drills for Civil Defense, driving a school bus, and nursing kidney dialysis patients. We follow in their footsteps with pride and gratitude.

Acknowledgement

This book respectfully acknowledges the millions of people who have lost their lives in natural or man-made disasters, and we honor them and the loved ones they left behind. We salute the courage and selflessness of the large numbers of the fallen who made the ultimate sacrifice or were injured or disabled helping others in a time of momentous crisis. We recognize the contribution of the professional emergency responders, military personnel, civic volunteers, and all the unsung heroes who rise up to meet the enormous challenges head on. The disaster survivors who joined their neighbors to rebuild in spite of catastrophic damages that stripped them of the most basic comforts must also be commended. Many special thanks to the grass roots efforts of emergency preparedness devotees who work hard every day to build better neighborhoods and resilient communities.

Authors Training

Emergency Management Institute
Homeland Security Evaluation Program, Volumes I, II, III
Federal Emergency Management Independent Study
   Courses:
   IS-00120.a Introduction to Exercises
   IS-00230.a Fundamentals of Emergency Management
   IS-00235.a Emergency Planning
   IS-00393.a Introduction to Hazard Mitigation
   IS-00630 Introduction to Public Assistance Process
   IS-00631 Public Assistance Operation I
Amateur Radio Licensee in Oregon for HAM radio
Neighborhood Emergency Team Leadership Course
Texas Engineering Extension Service in Cooperation with
   Dept. of Homeland Security and Federal Emergency
   Management Agency
Terrorist and Disaster Threat and Risk Assessment Course
Business Continuity Planning
Theory of Emergency Management

Regional Exercises
Washington County Civil Defense Fallout Shelter Nuclear
   Disaster Exercise
Washington County Full Scale Windstorm Exercise
Port of Portland Full Scale Aircraft Disaster Exercise
Portland Metro Region Cities Readiness Initiative Full
   Scale Pandemic Exercise
Oregon Shake-Out Earthquake Disaster Exercise
Plant Medicine & Disaster Herbalism Intensive Workshop

Contents

Preface: What You Will Learn from this Book 9
Introduction 13

General Preparation **17**
The Household Plan 21
Fire Drills 52
Utilities 58
Earthquake Drills 63
    Exterior Hazards 65
    Interior Hazards 71
After the Disaster Plan 77
Evacuation 83
Plans .88
    Insurance Company Plan 88
    Neighborhood Plan 99
    Pet Plan 102
    School Plan 104
    Workplace Plan 108
    Church Plan 111
    Bank Plan 113
    Retirement Facility Plan 114
Supplies Storage 118
List of Supplies to Store 120

Natural Disasters **131**
Earthquakes 133
Landslides 145
Tsunamis 151
Volcanic Eruptions 157
Hurricanes 165
Tornados 171

Floods. 179
Wildfires 185
Thunderstorms 193
Blizzards. 197
Cyclones. 203
Typhoons 207

Man-Made Disasters 211
Bombings and Explosions 213
Nuclear Occurrences 221
Toxic Chemical Releases 231
Power Outages 243

Communications in a Disaster 263

In Summary 273

Resource Guides
SmartPhone/Droid/iPad/iPod/iTunes 275
Recommended Websites 283
Recommended Books. 289

What You Will Learn from this Book

Our purpose in writing this book is to show individuals, households, and families how to prepare for natural and man-made disasters. **Every person alive today will likely face at least one natural disaster in their lifetime, and 60 to 70 percent of people will experience a serious trauma.** According to the American Red Cross, less than 10 percent of Americans are prepared for such a disaster. The consequence of not preparing can make the difference of mere seconds between life and death. To prepare for a disaster, do the following:

- Create a kit
- Devise a plan
- Increase your awareness

We offer guidelines to facilitate awareness and develop organizational, self-reliance, and survival skills. When a disaster hits, survival and quality of life will depend on your preparedness. Our main focus is to increase your awareness and prepare you for disasters that may happen to you, wherever you may be. Saving lives, minimizing injuries, lessening monetary and property damages, and coping successfully afterwards all depends on what is done beforehand. We will share with you historical information from worldwide disasters to new technologies that will propel you into a mindset of resilient thinking and action. Our number one recommendation: save yourself first. Otherwise, you will not be of any help to anyone else.

This book will educate you on the steps to take before, during, and after a disaster. Preparedness is critical in the event of any disaster and this book will allow you maximize your preparedness. The household or family plan will show you how to check your insurance coverage, inventory your possessions, and store important information. We will show you how to set up an out-of-area contact person and how to reunite with your family or household after a disaster. The school plan will provide questions to ask your children's schools, including the details of their emergency plans. The neighborhood plan will teach you how to strengthen your community. Building a resilient community that can bounce back from a disaster will help you, your family, and your general community plan for any disaster that could hit your geographic area.

This book will also offer resources for retrofitting, bracing, and sheathing your home and will address structural and safety hazards. We will provide detailed information on current smart phone applications that you can use to stay connected to your household or family members and your out-of-area contact person. You will also learn how to turn your cell phone into a radio, GPS tracking device, or medical encyclopedia including your own personal medical history. We will direct you to web-based tools for mapping and saving multiple escape routes. We will cover building a home-emergency kit and storing water, food, and supplies including first aid kits and pet kits. Separate emergency kit lists will also be provided for car, work, and school.

The general preparedness section provides organizational checklists for you to use before disaster strikes. We educate you on how to evaluate the prevailing conditions after the disaster and decide whether to evacuate or take shelter in your home. We'll also cover a broad scope of natural disasters from flooding to earthquakes and include new chapters on man-made disasters from toxic chemical spills to nuclear accidents. An introduction for each chapter will include a concise description and explanation of each event with examples of specific occurrences. We will discuss the predictability of disasters by season, historical occurrence, geographic region, and their warning systems.

Reading this book will greatly increase your odds of survival and quality of life following a natural or man-made disaster. Knowing what disasters you may face where you live or visit will frame your awareness. Read the chapters that apply to your area first, whether you are on the flood plain, in earthquake country, or near a nuclear power plant. Check our Resource Guide, located in the back of the book, to learn cell phone technology that you can use now, as well as how to utilize Google Maps to plan escape routes for you and your household, family, and friends. Our goal is to increase your situational awareness from this day forward.

Introduction

On March 11, 2011, a 9.0 magnitude earthquake upended the east coast of Japan and set off a 30-foot tsunami that swept away towns and set the stage for a meltdown of two nuclear power plants. The country was besieged by its worst seismic event of the century and two additional catastrophes. The year of 2010 had also seen unbridled natural and man-made disasters worldwide. Mine collapses, floods, earthquakes, and hurricanes were the worst on record. Learn more about some of the worst disasters in history (www.epicdisasters.com).

The long and colorful history of natural disasters is well documented. Scientific observations and studies are ongoing, but the phenomena they describe can't be directly altered or prevented. The weather is beyond human control. The barometric pressure, the velocity of the winds, and the humidity that make up the earth's atmosphere are way beyond the reach and regulation of mortal human beings. The orbit and rotation of the earth and its internal movements cannot be controlled. The shifting and colliding of the crust's massive continental plates is perpetual. The buildup of thermal pressures deep in the earth's core cannot be stopped from rising to a boil. Nature's turbulent forces will continue to manifest in disasters that burst on the scene anywhere and everywhere on the planet.

Enormous natural disasters are capable of kick-starting other disasters that bring on a double or even triple series of events with far-reaching affects and heavy tolls. The earthquake in Japan in 2011 triggered a tsunami that traveled over 5,000 miles by sea and put over 50 countries on tsunami alert before it powered into foreign coastlines. A year earlier, a violent magnitude 7.0 temblor struck Haiti on Jan. 12, 2010 and killed 230,000 people. The earth moved again and devastation spiraled out of control one short month later when an 8.8 magnitude quake rocked Chile's central coast on Feb. 27, 2010, killing more than 500 people. Fortunately property damage was minimized by the country's enforcement of stringent building codes. A catastrophic cyclone wrought massive damage in western Myanmar on Oct. 22, 2010, and a typhoon littered the Philippines with a wide trail of debris and destruction—including 100 fatalities. In July of the same year, heavy flooding submerged nearly a third of Pakistan in one of the world's worst natural disasters of all time. The United Nations (U.N.) estimated that as many as 21 million people lost their homes and over 1,700 died due to the July–August inundation.

The catastrophic drama of 2010 spread across the globe and hit the United States. The largest man-made disaster in the history of the petroleum industry sent crude oil spewing from a deep sea well into the Gulf of Mexico and into the mouth of the Mississippi River for over three months. The Deepwater Horizon blowout polluted the Gulf with 49 million barrels of raw petroleum before the leak was finally capped. Scientists' studies of the spill's pollution and its damage to marine and wildlife habitats are ongoing. Projections estimate that the adverse effects are likely to linger for decades. The economically essential Gulf fishing industry was crippled as well, and recovery may take a long time. Check online (www.earthweek.com) for reports and updates on affected wildlife and ecosystems.

We will cover the impact of man-made disasters and the tactics to survive them. Like natural disasters, man-made disasters strike suddenly and increase the state of emergency in any community, region, or country. These industrial level accidents occur randomly, outside the normal course of events. Enormous destruction and chaos can be caused by human error, mistakes in judgment, negligence, equipment failures, and mismanagement of inclement weather conditions. In addition, sudden accidents can happen anywhere hazardous materials are being stored or transported.

A deliberate attack, as in the use of chemical or biological weapons or cyber sabotage by terrorists, is also a possible danger. Over one million readers a month view this site (www.nationalterroralert.com) to check on possible worldwide terror events. The intentional release and infusion of chemicals or other hazardous materials into the environment is different from an accidental spill or leak, but preparedness for and response to either event is very similar. Being prepared for and knowing what to do in the event of an accidental chemical spill also allows one to be ready in the event of a terrorist attack.

The Importance of Psychological Care

Professor Edna Foe of the University of Pennsylvania states that once a disaster strikes, psychological care is an imperative part of recovery. *TIME magazine* named Edna Foe, PhD, to the *2010 TIME 100*, the magazine's annual list of the 100 most influential people in the world (http://www.uphs.upenn.edu/news/News_Releases/2010/04/ptsd-researcher-most-influential-time-magazine). In 2002, she reported that between eight and 10 percent of the population suffers from post-traumatic stress disorder (PTSD), and that one-third of those suffer symptoms 10 years *after* their first experience. You can access her extensive research and findings online (www.anxietystudycenter.org).

Massive PTSD symptoms have been documented in returning war vets and those experiencing extreme stress from disasters such as Hurricane Katrina and the Gulf oil spill. Treatment for survivors of disasters with PTSD involves learning coping strategies where therapists help redirect harmful thinking and "what if" scenarios, especially when he or she felt responsible for the ensuing tragedy. By preparing and being proactive, you can forestall the added development of deeper psychological problems, such as PTSD for yourself, your family, and your community. Survivor's stress is well documented through online sources (www.psychcentral.com).

Investigative journalist Amanda Ripley's book, *The Unthinkable: Who Survives When Disaster Strikes*, details what went on inside the heads of heroes and everyday people. It studies workers in the World Trade Center twin towers on 9/11, passengers caught aboard burning jet aircraft, and those thrown into icy rivers unexpectedly. Ripley conducts detailed interviews with survivors and reveals that their preparedness and situational awareness saved their lives. She also reveals details on the PTSD symptoms that survivors live with now. View Ripley's findings online (www.amandaripley.com).

When any natural or man-made disaster strikes, thousands to hundreds of thousands of people can be overwhelmed by the event at once. Rescue services and emergency responders will be overworked in the first seven days to three weeks of any disaster. Authorities say 9-1-1 call centers may not be able to answer all calls. For that reason, survival and relative quality of life will depend on your preparedness level and self-reliance. Being ready with stored supplies and advance training is the key, and can mean the difference between life and death.

General Preparation

Outdoor enthusiasts have long understood and followed common sense regimens to ensure survival in the wild. The Boy Scouts' famous motto is: "Be prepared." Campers and hikers practice basic safety and survival skills to anticipate possible problems and to be ready for changing conditions such as inclement weather, damaged equipment or watercraft, injuries to party members, or lost hikers. These rules can also apply in natural and man-made disasters. Experts agree that the best way to prepare for a disaster is to have a disaster plan. Preparedness is the key to meeting the challenge of any crisis event, whether it is a natural or man-made disaster.

As we've illustrated, disasters can hit suddenly and create wide-reaching distress and destruction. Prevention of disasters is not possible, but statistics show that advanced planning and development of survival skills *can* save lives. According to the International Committee of the Red Cross (ICRC), the odds of surviving any disaster dramatically increases with heightened levels of preparedness. Access the Red Cross's resources, quick links, and services online (www.icrc.org).

Sudden Events

It is very important to be ready to evacuate or get immediately to shelter if a disaster occurs. Once disaster strikes, there is no time to shop or search for supplies. Preparations against potential threats must be made in advance. A tornado or earthquake could hit with sudden force. A truck carrying toxic chemicals could overturn on the highway. A dam could burst. An outbreak of smallpox or botulism could strike without warning. A winter blizzard could stop a community in its tracks and leave hundreds or thousands of people confined to their homes without water, power, or telephones.

Self-Reliance

In a disaster, emergency responders, firefighters, paramedics, and police will be on the job; but all affected people cannot be reached at once. As mentioned previously, people may be on their own for anywhere from seven days to three weeks. Experts agree that self-reliance promotes survival. Blending a self-reliant approach into your daily life will create success for you and your household in responding to a disaster. At the core of good preparedness is the concept of taking responsibility for personal and family safety. Making a commitment to general preparedness is a positive and proactive approach no matter where you live or travel.

From this basic commitment, building a household plan and a disaster kit is the next step. Basic components of a well-stocked emergency kit include adequate water, food, and supplies to allow for sustainability after a disaster. Building the kit involves simple organizational tasks of gathering canned goods and bottled water, rounding up camping supplies and flashlights, and collecting a first aid kit with spare prescription glasses and medications. Conducting regular fire and evacuation drills will train household and family members to develop correct responses to prevailing threats, and these learned actions will then kick in automatically in the event of a real emergency. Being ready for any emergency of any scope, from a fire to an earthquake, makes good, common sense. Other preparedness components that we'll cover are CPR training, Neighborhood Emergency Team (NET or CERT) training, and Red Cross first aid classes (see www.citizenscorp.gov/cert). The CPR method is updated regularly, and there are new techniques being taught community-wide as well as pet CPR skills. View the Heart Association video and website for more details (http://handsonlycpr.org).

As practice drills are conducted, simple habits and survival skills will be cultivated and melded into your everyday life. By following our guidelines, your survival skills will become like second nature. For example, keeping the car's gasoline tank filled and bottled water in the trunk will be automatic. Driving alternative routes to destinations will be a painless way to become more aware of nearby surroundings and prepare for evacuation. Looking for emergency exits in a theatre, stadium, or airport will become effortless with repetition. These daily preparation actions are easy and undeniably necessary for disaster survival.

Information Gathering and Organization

Information gathering and organization is a basic step in good preparedness. Documentation and itemization of household possessions, valuables and collectables, family heirlooms, insurance policies, and financial records is central to emergency planning. In case of any insurance claims, the paperwork will need to be in order and accessible. Photographs and sales receipts will prove the existence and value of property and furnishings when damage or loss occurs.

A thorough household inventory that is updated annually protects your assets. Document any additions that add protection to your home such as alarm systems, sprinkler systems, and other safety measures for possible premium discounts. Insurance policies, important papers and records, and other valuables can be placed in a safe deposit box. Belongings with sentimental value like favorite family photos can be copied on a CD or a backup digital disk for storage. Online resources (www.knowyourstuff.org) can help you organize your possessions. Include copies of everything mentioned above in your emergency kit. As a backup, you also can send copies of photos and important information to an out-of-area contact person.

In addition, consider meeting with your insurance agent annually for a review of your policies and coverage. Be sure to document any improvements or renovations made to the house in your updated inventory. Exterior decking or a new family room could add value to your home. Adding sprinkler systems and monitored alarm systems may also bring insurance discounts. Reviewing and updating household inventories and increasing insurance coverage could very well be money in the bank later. For example, if there is a flood or fire, you would want to be reimbursed for the additional value of the $50,000 kitchen remodel you had done last year.

In addition, you'll want to prepare beyond the home. Information gathering on community preparedness, emergency warning systems, neighborhood watch groups and associations, and emergency shelters or staging areas is important. Also, contact children's schools and grandparent's nursing homes for information on fire drills, emergency plans, and evacuation procedures. Similar inquiries can be made at the workplace and at your church.

Household Walk Through

Individuals living alone, roommates, and families should all conduct a walk through outside and inside of the home. You can do this by creating a list of disaster preparedness steps such as bracing chimneys, shoring up weak roof lines, meeting seismic codes, securing or bolting down heavy furniture, cleaning up storage areas, and cutting brush away from the house. Go to the Federal Emergency Management Agency (FEMA) website (www.fema.gov) to learn about various types of hazards. Designate safe places to take cover during a disaster and emergency exits. Map out and draw an escape route for your home and work. After testing fire extinguishers and smoke alarms, conduct fire drills and

General Preparation

other emergency exercises. Write down a plan and discuss it with your family or household members. You will want to re-evaluate the plan every three to six months.

The Household Plan

Preparedness has been statistically proven to save lives, lessen trauma, minimize injuries, and reduce property damage. The household plan is the most basic and important step to prepare for any disaster that you and your loved ones face. It is a form of insurance that will promote necessary mental, emotional, and physical readiness for any disaster that may occur. Single member households, roommates, couples, and families can all benefit by creating a household plan. Walk through the colorful and fun FEMA for Kids site (www.fema.gov/kids) where you can play games with youngsters as you establish the importance of a household or family plan, the need for two escape routes, and learn how to create emergency kits. By working and training together as a unit, your household will be able to take control in a crisis.

Reflect on the specific threats you face geographically and seasonally in your area, and prepare for them. If you are in earthquake country, as many regions are, prepare for an earthquake. Other events can be more predictable. Seasonal hurricanes, wildfires, tornados, thunderstorms, or blizzards can often be forecast. When an unpredicted man-made calamity strikes, your household plan will make you ready for it as well. Review the plan annually to reassess household needs, insurance coverage, financial information, and medical data. Update emergency supply kits with fresh water, food, flashlight batteries, seasonal clothing, prescription medications, and eyeglasses. Having a good general preparation plan is an ongoing process—one that you can update regularly (every three to six months).

Household Meeting

The time to devise an emergency plan is long before a disaster occurs, catching everyone off guard. Calling a household or family meeting is the first step. Everyone in the household should be included in the discussion. Pick someone to be in charge and a back-up commander so everyone knows who to turn to first and second when disaster strikes. Evaluating potential dangers, planning escape routes, choosing safe places to shelter or meet later, and gathering supplies and important papers are all elements of overall preparedness. Map your routes and save them to Google Maps where you can share the data virtually with your household, family, and out-of-area contact person.

A household plan is the blueprint of emergency operations, and should start first with a simple drawing of the house floor plan, including two possible exits from every room. Locations of fire extinguishers, emergency and first aid kits, gas, electric and water shutoffs, and special equipment like rope ladders and chainsaws should all be noted in the house drawing. Decide on a place to meet outside of the house that is a safe distance away in case of fire, flood, or structural damage. Pick a meeting place outside of the neighborhood in case returning home is not possible. Utilize web mapping techniques for designing rendezvous points after a disaster. Save these to your cell phone, computer tablets, and iPods.

Parents should make backup child care arrangements in case they cannot return home. Children may need to stay at school or with neighbors or relatives. Hurricane Katrina left over 5,000 children without a parent due to evacuations. The Center for Missing and Exploited Children (www.missingkids.com) and the Red Cross (www.familylinks.icrc.org) brought all of those children back together with their families, but it took several months. Both organizations do extensive work in a disaster area to register and reunite children. After the March 11, 2011 earthquake in Japan normal communications channels were down, but Google set up a site where families and others could search over the Internet for those lost in the affected area (http://japan.person-finder.appspot.com/?lang=en). A visitor can enter information (in over seven languages) about someone they are looking for or someone they have found.

Web-based applications and cloud management of data from disaster areas is gaining worldwide attention. The Google Crisis Response Project stepped up in disasters all over the globe, from the horrific devastation in New Orleans during Hurricane Katrina to the earthquakes in Chile, New Zealand, and Japan. Google opened up satellite images, news alerts, and even donation options without sensationalist reporting, and offered a way to track people down in a disaster. In Haiti, facial software recognition programs were developed by computer programmers and application geeks worldwide to help identify lost individuals. This innovative web-based response from volunteers worldwide has forever changed and improved emergency responses for the future. Learn how this is changing the response to disasters worldwide (http://www.google.com/crisisresponse).

Out-of-Area Emergency Contact Person

When disaster strikes, contacting other household and family members is a paramount concern. However, communication vehicles may not cooperate. Local telephone circuits may be overloaded. Landlines and cell phones may only work intermittently. Disaster authorities say text messaging was highly used after recent tragedies in Japan, Haiti, and Chile. Knowing how to text a message before a disaster will help you become more resilient in the chaos of disasters when local phone lines are overwhelmed. Fortunately, phone companies will sometimes free up long distance lines, making long distance service one of the most viable communication options. Because of this, emergency responders and disaster experts recommend choosing someone who lives in another state as your contact person. Phone apps also exist that can capture your location and upload it to your emergency contacts through cloud computing, using remote computers rather than having to input via a personal computer.

Please note: It will serve you well to test and use your communication device(s) and any applications *before* a disaster strikes. Once you upload a phone application, practice using it to retrieve or send information to other household members and your out-of-area contact person. Practice using Twitter or logging into Facebook or other social media sites. Don't wait until a disaster strikes to do it for the first time. Check the Resource Guide in the back of this book for detailed information on related phone applications and websites to find out how you can listen to social media conversations by using Hootsuite and Tweetdeck for updated weather tips, current trends, and breaking news. Disaster scene data is always available with eyewitness reporting that includes pictures and videos. The National Weather Service and FEMA post updates to Twitter, Facebook, and YouTube and disseminate information in this way during disasters. Learning the appropriate technology now allows you to receive the most real-time updates in a disaster.

Make an agreement in advance with a friend or relative who will store your important medical, insurance, legal, and financial information, and act as a message center. He or she should be far enough away to be unaffected by your disaster. If you do not have an out-of-area contact person, you can also consider storing your personal medical data in a folder on your refrigerator. Firefighters and first responders are trained to look on top of the refrigerator for this information and to also look through your cell phone for your emergency contacts, medical information, and prescription medications. However, this will only be helpful in the event that your home is not destroyed in some way.

The contact person will serve three purposes. First, he or she can relay information about the well-being and location of household and family members to others who may have lost touch during the disaster. This will help everyone know where and when it is safe to reunite. Second, the contact will store copies of photographs, important records, and documents on email, CDs, and flash drives which can be sent as needed. Third, the contact will provide rescue and medical personnel, as well as insurance representatives with vital statistics and information. Maintain your emergency contacts in your cell phone through the ICE (In Case of Emergency) cell phone application and other emergency applications (see Resource Guide). A free tool for national disasters is the Next Of Kin Registry (NOKR) (http://www.nokr.org). This central emergency contact system is a nonprofit organization whose mission is to bring you and your household together—whether nationally or internationally—when injured, missing, or deceased. Once you register, stored information is secured. NOKR is used in the United States and in over 85 countries.

In a life and death emergency, the contact person could act on your behalf as your personal representative with Medical Power of Attorney. He or she can forward a copy of your last will, signed medical releases, directives to physicians and vital information on everyone and give surviving heirs necessary legal, banking, business, real estate, and insurance documents. It is imperative that you carry critical medical information with you if possible. There are phone apps that can help you organize this info and make it accessible when you need it. Check the Resource Guide at the end of this book for a list of applications for various phone types.

Below is a suggested list of information to provide to your out-of-area contact person so they can act on your behalf in case of a disaster. Be sure to include the contact person's name, address, telephone number, cell phone number, and email address. Important phone numbers can be stored on a postcard size laminated sheet, kept in wallets or backpacks, in vehicles, in the emergency kit, and forwarded to the contact by mail or email. A hard copy of this list and original documents can be included in a safe deposit box. Also, keep a copy in your emergency supply kit (more detailed information on putting this together to follow). A copy can be mailed to the contact person or scanned into the computer and emailed. It can also be saved on a CD or flash drive for more compact and efficient storage and portability.

Children's Data (update annually)
- Full names and birth date
- Cell phone numbers
- Social security numbers
- Color of eyes and hair
- Sex and race
- Height and weight
- Any scars, birthmarks, or other distinguishing physical characteristics
- Other identifiers such as glasses, braces, broken arm, etc.
- Daycare or school name, address, phone number, contact person, cell, and email
- Pediatrician/physician and phone number(s)
- Signed medical releases

- Immunization records
- Recent surgeries and hospitalizations
- Copy of fingerprints and current photographs
- Copy of passports
- Babysitter's name and phone number
- Blood type and allergies
- Special medical conditions, handicaps, medical equipment, etc.
- Regular prescription medications and pharmacy contact phone number
- Name of adult (not a parent) to pick up child, password to use and cell phone number

Adult's Data
- Full names and birth dates
- Home, work, cell phone numbers, email address
- Home address
- Social security numbers
- Family physician, office phone number, cell phone
- Signed medical releases
- Advance directives to physicians
- Immunization records, recent surgeries
- Preferred hospital, name, address, phone number, email
- Pharmacy name, address, phone number, 24-hour numbers
- List of regular prescription medications
- Medical policies and cards
- Blood type and allergies
- Special health problems, handicaps, medical equipment, etc.
- Person(s) to notify in an emergency, phone numbers, cell phone numbers, emails
- Religious preferences

Children's Data

Name: _____

Gender: _____ Height: _____ Weight: _____

Address: _____

City/State/Zip: _____

Home Phone: _____ Cell Phone: _____

Blood Type: _____

Allergies: _____

Date of Birth: _____

SS#: _____

Daycare or Sitter: _____

Address: _____

City/State/Zip: _____

Home Phone: _____ Cell Phone: _____

Next of Kin: _____

Emergency Information

In-Area Contact Person: _____

Out-of-Area Contact Person: _____

School Address: _____

City/State/Zip: _____

Phone: _____ Email: _____

Google-groups List: _____ Twitter: _____

Phone: _____

Text Message: _____ Other: _____

Medical Conditions: _____

Prescriptions: _____

Doctor: _____ Phone: _____

Doctor: _____ Phone: _____

Insurance: _____

Adult's Data

Name: _____

Gender: _____ Height: _____ Weight: _____

Address: _____

City/State/Zip: _____

Home Phone: _____ Cell Phone: _____

Blood Type: _____

Allergies: _____

Date of Birth: _____

SS#: _____

Bank: _____ Phone: _____

Insurance contact: _____ Phone: _____

Attorney: _____ Phone: _____

Next of Kin: _____

Emergency Information

In-Area Contact Person: _____

Out-of-Area Contact Person: _____

Address: _____

City/State/Zip: _____

Home Phone: _____ Cell Phone: _____

Notification by Facebook: _____

Google-groups List: _____ Twitter: _____

Phone: _____

Text Message: _____ Other: _____

Medical Conditions: _____

Prescriptions: _____

Doctor: _____ Phone: _____

Doctor: _____ Phone: _____

Insurance: _____

Legal and Business Records
　Attorney or executor's names, office and cell phone numbers, e-mail address
　Power of Attorney
　Bank name, branch address, contact person, phone number, and email
　Checking account number
　Savings account or Certificate of Deposit number
　Savings bonds
　Credit card companies, account numbers, phone numbers, emails, websites
　Stocks and bonds, broker, office phone, cell phone, email
　Safety deposit box number, bank, address (include copy of the key in the parcel)
　Mortgage company, account number, phone number, email, website
　Mortgage deed
　Patents, copyrights, and trademarks
　Recent personal and business tax records, 2 years for self-employed people

Personal Papers, Household and Family Records
　Marriage certificate, divorce decree
　Death certificate
　Diplomas
　Passport, Visa, driver's license copies
　Auto, boat and RV titles, bills of sale, license numbers, VIN numbers
　Auto insurance policy, office phone, agent name, cell phone, email
　Homeowners insurance company, policy number, agent name, office phone, cell Inventory of household goods and valuables

Life insurance carrier, policy number, agent name, office phone, cell phone, email
Photographs and digital SD cards or CDs
Naturalization papers
Military papers and discharges
Copy of last will

Jewelry and Collectables
Heirloom possessions
Precious metals and coins
Medals
Stamps
Rare artifacts

Supply Gathering and Building Emergency Kits

Make supply gathering a household project similar to getting gear together for a camping or backpacking excursion. Together, you will help build your emergency disaster kit. Select a spot to store the kit where it is safe, accessible, cool, and dry. This could be in a garage, storage shed, or basement. Round up or buy a container for the emergency supplies like a rolling duffle bag or a large garbage can on wheels with a secure lid. Water should be stored separately where it can't leak on clothing or bedding.

Supply contents should include:
- One gallon of water per person, per day for drinking and washing.
- A three-day to three-week supply of nonperishable food.
- Canned goods and dehydrated meals that you have tried and like.
- Dated food, water, and other perishables. Check and refresh every six months.
- Consider any food allergies when packing foods.

- ❏ Add first aid supplies along with a Red Cross instruction manual.
- ❏ Include prescription medications, personal hygiene items, and extra prescription eyeglasses.
- ❏ Pack special medical items such as syringes and blood pressure monitors.
- ❏ Pull together camping equipment, tent, sleeping bags, pads, chairs, propane stoves, flashlights, and lanterns. Rotate and replace supplies as necessary.
- ❏ Stock a portable radio for receiving the most accurate and timely disaster warnings, advisements, and evacuation information.
- ❏ Store batteries for radio and other electronic items separately or secure them to the radio casing with duct or electrical tape.
- ❏ Find Emergency Broadcast System radios, crank radios, and solar powered radios and cell phone chargers that don't need batteries online and read user reviews before purchasing.

Once the main disaster kit is built, other smaller versions of emergency kits can be assembled. Put mini emergency kits under everyone's bed for quick access at night. For traveling, put kits in all vehicles, RVs, and boats. Schools are now aware of the need for children to have an emergency kit available to them at school. Ask your school administrator if your school has a plan and kits with water and food for children who may be trapped by a disaster for hours or days. Ask if you can personalize kits already prepared by adding photos, a cuddle buddy, or favorite toy. Also, prepare an office kit to keep at work. Make a kit for your pet(s) too. Kits are available online for home, office, and school, and for cats and dogs. Check our website for a recommended source for regular emergency

General Preparation

supplies (www.naturaldisastersbook.com). You can pur kosher emergency kits to meet special needs (www.prepared.com).

Under the Bed Emergency Kit

Most people sleep an average of eight hours a night, and about a third of every 24-hour period is spent in bed. Therefore, the risk of a disaster hitting while you are sleeping is roughly 33 percent. According to the United States government one-stop fire safety information online resource in English and Spanish (www.FireSafety.gov), residential fires accounted for 85 percent of all fire deaths in 2009. In addition, from 2000–2009 an average of 2,919 civilians lost their lives and 14,081 suffered injuries from home fires—most of which occurred at night. These risks are high enough to warrant being prepared and making sure you and your household are safe. That way, if you're suddenly awakened by a disaster, you'll be ready. Following the content list below, have everyone create an emergency kit to keep under their bed. Contain supplies in a small box, gym bag, or backpack.

Contents of an under the bed emergency kit:
- ❑ Include a teddy bear, doll, or other favorite cuddle buddy for small children.
- ❑ Pack a flashlight to find your way in the dark and see obstacles in your path.
- ❑ Add heavy shoes and socks that will protect your feet and get you through mud, debris, or broken glass.
- ❑ Include practical, seasonal clothing that will protect arms and legs. Sweat clothes, a hat or skullcap, a plastic poncho or a parka with a hood, even a black plastic trash bag will keep you dry.

- ❑ Pack heavy work gloves to protect your hands and enable debris clearing, like picking up broken glass and other tasks.
- ❑ Include a crank cell phone charger to enable communication and receive disaster updates and alerts. Keep your cell phone handy.
- ❑ Add a small portable radio for breaking news reports, alerts, and instructions. Keep batteries separate.
- ❑ Include a jug of water for drinking and washing off.
- ❑ In case of a fire, have a towel to wet down and stick under the bedroom door to keep smoke away or to hold over your nose and mouth as you exit.
- ❑ Include a rope ladder for escape from a second story bedroom.

Whether escaping a fire, sheltering from a tornado inside or reacting to any other sudden emergency, you will be ready.

Storing Supplies for the Disaster Kit

Once the supplies are stored and kits are built, it's time to designate household and family responsibilities and duties in the event of a disaster. Post duties on a bulletin board or refrigerator with a dated checklist of who will be responsible for what. Include younger children by having them help put together their under the bed kits and choose a favorite stuffed animal or doll. This gets them involved and is something you can all share together.

If you have pets, call local shelters, motels, and hotels to find out if they will take pets as well as the limits on breed, size, and number of animals. Talk to local veterinarians about sheltering pets and recommended boarding kennels. If advance warning permits, call for reservations. Always be sure to leave written permission and instructions for a neighbor to care for pets while you are away.

General Preparation 35

Other actions to take:
- ❏ Talk to your local pharmacist about safe storage of medicines.
- ❏ Copy car and house keys at a locksmith or hardware store and keep in designated hiding places and emergency kits. Also, hide one house key outside in an agreed upon spot.
- ❏ Store shutoff tools at the gas meter, near the water main, and keep a spare tool in your disaster kit in case you need to help others. Review detailed instructions on shutoff techniques online (www.fema.gov/plan/prepare/utilityplan.shtm).
- ❏ Only shut off your gas if you smell a leak. Be aware that gas utility companies warn against turning off your gas because you will have to wait for technicians to turn the service back on. If you shut off your gas or water, be prepared to evacuate in the event of no heat or water.
- ❏ Store flashlights and spare batteries on each floor by exits and in disaster kits.
- ❏ Buy smoke alarms and install them near every bedroom and on each floor of the house.
- ❏ Install Carbon Monoxide alarms to warn you of odorless, poisonous CO gas.
- ❏ Buy and learn to operate ABC fire extinguishers, and test every six months.
  - Store firefighting tools, equipment and hoses in one place.
- ❏ Contact the fire department for a hazards list, fire drill information, and safety tips or look online (www.usfa.dhs.gov/citizens/home_fire_prev).
- ❏ Conduct regular fire drills. Practice at home with all members of the household.

- ❑ Write up a list of emergency numbers and tape it to every telephone in the house.
- ❑ Use a phone app to highlight and store numbers in your mobile phones.
  - Check the Resource Guide at the end of the book for more cell phone applications for emergency preparedness.
- ❑ Learn how to use text messaging on cell phones to bypass overloaded phone networks.
  - Check with your service provider on advance sign-ups and fees. Be sure everyone is trained on how to do this.
- ❑ Use ICE (see Resource Guide) on all of your cell phones.
- ❑ Learn how to manually override the cell phone network and use roaming to utilize other cellular networks that may not be jammed.
- ❑ Research emergency communications and hand-held email and wireless Internet devices like RIM Blackberry, and wireless Internet devices that worked after 9/11 and are used by the United States Congress.
- ❑ Research flood, earthquake, or other disaster insurance and obtain coverage.
- ❑ Store a copy of your insurance policy in your kit.
- ❑ Perform a household inventory of possessions and valuables. Visit the free insurance industry site and check the Resource Guide at the end of the book for more details (www.knowyourstuff.org).
- ❑ Check and replace flashlight and radio batteries.
- ❑ Take photographs or videos of belongings, and valuables for insurance inventory. Install digital photos on your computer and email to your out-of-area contact person.
- ❑ Gather documents to copy and store in a safe

General Preparation 37

deposit box. Copy to a removable disk and email the information to your out-of-area contact person, and keep copies of the following in emergency kits:
- Social Security card(s)
- Driver's licenses, passports, birth certificates
- Marriage certificates, death certificates
- Probate files and wills
- Contracts, mortgage statements, deeds
- Stocks and bonds
- Bank account numbers, savings account numbers, Certificate of Deposit numbers
- Credit card companies and account numbers, PIN numbers or codes
- Insurance policies
- Immunization and vaccination records
- Medical Power of Attorney

Personal Medical Information for Disaster Kits

List all household and family members on a red medical emergency card to display on the refrigerator. If paramedics come, they will be able to access the essential information. Include the following:
- ❏ Blood type
- ❏ Allergies
- ❏ Medical conditions for everyone
- ❏ Dialysis schedule
- ❏ Heart patient care medications
- ❏ Diabetic levels and drugs used
- ❏ Seizure disorder
- ❏ High blood pressure medications
- ❏ Chemical sensitivities
- ❏ Physician's names and phone numbers
- ❏ Prescription medications, recent surgeries

- ❑ "Do Not Resuscitate" orders (DNR)
- ❑ Physician order for life sustaining treatment (Healthcare Directive)
- ❑ Emergency contact names with phone and cell phone numbers

Information Gathering and Education

Information gathering and education are critical tools in managing emergency preparedness because understanding diffuses fear, reduces apprehension, and makes coping easier. Panic reactions triggered by a larger than life event deter the ability to make correct survival decisions. It is empowering to think through the possible scenarios ahead of time and plan what the best actions are. Follow and discuss newspaper and television accounts of local or worldwide disasters to increase your family's awareness and familiarity levels.

Make sure that everyone who comes to your home is shown where emergency kits are stored. Show the babysitter, the housekeeper, and the caregiver where the disaster kit is located and run through the emergency plan, including fire exits and drills, where to shelter in place, and emergency cell phone numbers. Also provide the out-of-area contact name and telephone number. Share this information with houseguests and visitors as well.

Practice seasonal disaster drills throughout the year. Rotate food and water stock using products before they become outdated. Practice preparing an emergency meal with rotating stock. Make a dinner from your food inventory under the best-case scenario to see if you like what you're storing. You can also follow the award-winning program developed by LuAn Johnson, PhD, to Map Your Neighborhood (http://www.emd.wa.gov/myn/index.shtml).

Make a list of ill or disabled neighbors with special needs. Contact neighbors to develop a support system and a neighborhood plan. For details on how to establish a neighborhood response effort with Mapping Your Neighborhood go online (www.emd.wa.gov). Another program from this area is Seattle Neighborhoods Actively Prepare (SNAP). For instructions on how to get your neighborhood organized, check online (www.seattle.gov/emergency/programs/snap). Multiple languages translations are also available in this program.

Disasters to Anticipate
At the household meeting, discuss what types of disasters could happen in your area or where you will be traveling. Some disasters can happen anywhere and others are geographically specific. Fire is a possibility anywhere, but volcanic eruptions are not. Some disasters are seasonal; tropical storms like hurricanes and cyclones can be anticipated in certain months of the year. There are phone apps that store multiple disaster plans for you if you live in areas that are subject to flooding, earthquakes, tsunamis, or wildfires.

Thunderstorms are common all over the world. They happen almost everywhere, producing a wide range of threats. Lightning strikes, tornadoes, hailstorms, turbulent winds, and flash flooding all begin as thunderstorms. It is important to research the area you're traveling to or where you currently live to find out what types of natural disasters are possible. This will make your emergency plan much more strategic. Also, see the Resource Guide for suggested phone apps for early warning travel alerts.

Warning Systems
Communities rely on emergency warning systems to understand what is happening. Fire bells, foghorns, and sirens all carry different meanings and signal different actions. Education on community warning systems is critical in responding

to danger. If the fog horn signals a tsunami coming onto shore, evacuation would follow immediately, and residents schooled in the warning system would run to the highest ground. Teach children how to identify various warning system sounds. Listen to the sirens, foghorns, and church bells together and talk about what to do when they go off.

If you live in hurricane country, watch videos on tropical storms and hurricane alerts together. Discuss when to pick up the emergency kit and evacuate, and when to take cover in the basement and stay. Install and test smoke alarms in the house and let toddlers watch while older children act as helpers. Get everyone familiar with the sound of a smoke detector going off and how to react. Be proactive by working with neighborhood and community groups to test emergency warning equipment and alarms, warning horns, and emergency sirens. Have children participate with you, so they too become familiar with these various alarms.

Some warnings are expressed at varying levels of danger. Hurricane warnings are a good example. Pre-storm alerts broadcast on the radio and television using specific language: "Small Craft Warning," "Gale Warning," "Hurricane Watch," and "Hurricane Warning." The storm begins with a small craft warning, and then increases in seriousness until it escalates to a full hurricane warning. Know your surroundings. Be aware of natural hazards no matter where you are, and if you carry a cell phone utilize POM (Peace of Mind) Alerts that tune you into important public alerts by GPS location. In the United States, this links you to 19 government databases where you can customize alerts from Homeland Security to FEMA. Additional information is available at POM Alert Systems (http://govision2020.com/pomalerts.html). See the Resource Guide at end of book for more details on this phone app and others.

POM Alerts track National Weather, Homeland Security, and FEMA alerts which can be sent to your phone in seconds after they occur whether it is a tornado warning, icy roads, flood alert, or a threat to Homeland Security. Be aware that the local public alert systems are often preprogrammed from phone company records. This means if you do not have a published landline some phone companies will require you to register to be contacted—especially if you have a phone through a cable TV carrier. Check city or county government offices or websites to register your email address, cell phone, Internet phone, or landline phone from a cable carrier to receive alerts. On a National level, emergency and evacuation plans for man-made disasters are regulated by FEMA. Relevant information on preparedness, warning systems, and evacuation plans are available to the public via the FEMA website as well as educational materials and brochures. Check online (www.fema.gov) for more details.

Researching Preparedness Plans

Designate a household or family member to research disasters likely to affect your area through various agencies such as the Red Cross, FEMA, the Weather Bureau, and local emergency management. Get preparedness guides on each threat, including brochures and evacuation information from localized threats such as nuclear or chemical plants. Synch up with everyone using cell phone apps for early warning alerts, evacuation plans, and for storing records of prescription medications and surgical history. Local Amateur Radio clubs are also involved in emergency response. Check for these resources in your area. See the Resource Guide at the end of the book for more details. Discussing warning systems and learning the signals ahead of time is the most proactive way to be prepared for any disaster.

Threats to health also need to be considered. Recently, news all over the world has covered several deadly viruses such as Sudden Acute Respiratory Syndrome (SARS). SARS spread rapidly and killed hundreds of people from China to Toronto. Learn more details on worldwide disease threats (www.cdc.gov/sars). The West Nile Virus, transmitted by mosquito bites, has also been a major World Health Organization concern. Get a list of diseases likely to affect your community from your local health department. Being aware of health risks, prevention techniques, symptoms to watch for, and available treatment is important for good general preparedness. View up-to-date information on health risks worldwide (www.cdc.gov). You can read about public health emergencies, and how to respond to protect and save your life.

After the household and family are up to speed on general preparation techniques, open up a question and answer session so that everyone can participate. Make sure to have informational brochures available or have the websites mentioned previously on the computer for everyone to view. Broaden the household's education by visiting the library together to read more on natural and man-made threats. Being informed on the history and causes of both natural and man-made disasters can provide tremendous perspective for everyone.

School Studies

Children will likely study everything from earthquakes and storms (like tornados and hurricanes) in their science classes to more advanced courses that cover man-made disasters. To get an idea of the types of topics covered in science courses, go online (www.windows2universe.org) to National Earth Sciences teacher's lesson postings on earth movements in English and Spanish, and at three levels (beginner, intermediate, advanced). Children also learn about world history, and religious and economic differences that cause wars. While current events and political science classes will cover modern day terrorism, the book, *Terrorism and Kids* by Fern Reiss discusses how to talk to children about such threats. You can find this book online (www.terrorismandkids.com).

Involve the whole household in discussing historical disasters, including what is happening now and what could happen in the future. Talk about how to prepare for disasters, and answer any questions that may come up. Have children participate in emergency practice drills at school and share the techniques at home to ensure everyone is trained. Parents helping with drills at home will also reinforce the school's training.

Go online (www.fema.gov/kids) for teaching tools to help kids understand a disaster drill. The key is developing resilience in the face of any disaster. The more we practice, the better equipped we are to deal with our emotions during this critical time. Visit the Center for Disease Control and Prevention website (www.cdc.gov) for detailed help in talking with children from grade school to high school age about common reactions to disasters, and how to cope. The Red Cross is also a good source for taking care of your emotional health in a disaster (www.redcross.org). If you don't have Internet access and you have been in a disaster, you can call 1-866-GET-INFO to register yourself and your household members, and let others know about your welfare.

CPR and First Aid Training

It is said that 100,000 lives could be saved annually by proper application of CPR. Have at least one household or family member enroll in a CPR and first aid class at the YMCA, Red Cross, American Heart Association, or community center. Preparedness and emergency training classes and workshops are held in schools and churches as well. Emergency preparedness videos are available for checkout at local Red Cross sites and online (www.redcross.org). Watch these videos together as a household and then open up a discussion about what everyone learned. This will give children an opportunity to express fears, ask questions, and reduce anxieties by discussing what could happen and what can be done before, during, and after a disastrous event. CPR skills will prove useful in many different places and circumstances, at home or when traveling.

Children's Safety and Preparedness

There is always the possibility that a child could become separated from the rest of the family when shopping at the supermarket, on the way to school, or in a disaster; and there are steps to take ahead of time to reduce this stress.

- ❑ Set limits and establish neighborhood boundaries in which children are allowed to play.
- ❑ Stress good communication and insist on knowing where children will be.
- ❑ Establish time limits and curfews. Have children call home with updates on plans or times to return home.
- ❑ Early on, teach children their personal information. Help them memorize their name, address, home phone number, parents' work phone numbers, cell phone numbers, and email addresses as soon as possible. Knowing the name and phone numbers of the out-of-area contact person will link children with the rest of the household or family in an emergency.
- ❑ Giving older children a pre-paid phone card or a cell

phone will ensure that they can make and receive necessary calls.

Children's Identification

If a child is lost or missing, a detailed physical description can help find him/her. Being aware of your child's attire every day will aid police officials in their search. Current photographs of those missing can be shown around, given to police, and broadcast on television. New technology and legislation has established Amber Alerts using interstate computer systems and highway signs to greatly broaden the effort and success rate of finding missing children. Children's identification (I.D.) bracelets can be found online (www.mypreciouskid.com and www.kidsvitalids.com). Keep an up-to-date photo with your child's age, height, and weight on the back. Very young children can carry I.D. cards or bracelets. Be sure to give copies to babysitters or daycare workers. Parents' office and cell phone numbers and the out-of-area contact's phone numbers should be included on the I.D. cards. Also list blood types, allergies, and medications. Check with your local sheriff's office for free fingerprinting for children.

Getting Help

Act out scenarios together to teach children when to call for help. Read first-hand accounts of children as young as four years of age using this technique to save lives (www.yellandtell.com). Children learn who to ask for assistance with this method. Conduct rehearsals and take children to the supermarket, train station, shopping mall, or downtown. Teach children how to say "No!" to any stranger approaching them or trying to pull them into a car. Coach them to act aggressively in response to unwanted advances. Yell and tell tactics are supported by the following groups:

Girl and Boy Scouts
Camp Counselors
4-H Youth Leaders
Boys and Girls Club leaders
Kiwanis Key Clubs
Circle K Clubs
Youth Service Clubs
YMCA Youth Leaders
Church Youth Leaders

Encouraging children to trust any uneasy feelings in a situation can benefit them greatly. If a child comes home and thinks something doesn't look or feel right, let them know that they should go to a neighbor's house to get help. Become familiar with neighboring families and establish cooperative relations ahead of time. Make it easy for your child to seek help next door or down the block.

Passwords and Regular Routes

Agree on a password to use in case a designated adult other than a parent has to pick a child up from school, the airport, softball practice, the dentist, or church. Rehearse routes to and from regular destinations like school, friend's houses, playing fields, and community centers. Along the way, point out safe places to take cover and where to use the telephone. Conduct spot checks to make sure children are following the planned routes.

Calling 9-1-1

Explain when to call 9-1-1 and other emergency numbers for doctors, hospitals, and the out-of-area contact person. Go over what information to give when making emergency calls. Show children how to use phones and have them practice making calls. Show them cell phone operations, leaving and retrieving messages, and sending or retrieving email. At home, pre-program phones with one-touch emergency numbers for quick dialing. On a list that you keep near the phone, put parents' cell phone and office numbers, including the out-of-area contact's phone number. Update your child's cell phone with emergency numbers (ICE app—see Resource Guide and www.ice4safety.com to learn more about ICE).

Children's Emotional Needs

Children need guidance on how to prepare for a disaster as well as how to respond during and after. The National Association of School Psychologists breaks down the unique issues and coping challenges for children on their website by disaster type (www.nasponline.org). Schools are thought to be a vital player in helping kids cope with disasters by providing a familiar and safe environment after a disaster. Studies of children who have been through a natural disaster often show them with post-traumatic stress disorder (PTSD) even a year after the event. Learn more online about how PTSD can manifest in children who have experienced recent hurricanes (www.psychcentral.com).

It is important to understand how powerfully children are affected by these types of dramatic events. Establishing goals for reuniting after a disaster and getting to a new "normal" will help make children feel safe and well organized. Knowing what to expect and learning what to do will give them a feeling of control and balance. Helping alleviate their anxieties before a crisis event will enable them to cope better.

Children's Jobs

Children can participate in many different ways during disaster preparation. Help young children pack their under the bed emergency kits and add a cuddle buddy like a teddy bear. Prepare them for a possible separation by explaining that if you are away from home when something happens, you will return as soon as it is safe. Tuck a family snapshot into the kit, along with other small mementos that they choose. Helping gather and store household emergency supplies, building pet emergency kits and school kits are organizational jobs children can do. Education is a job too. Let children go to the library or Red Cross with you to pick out educational videos to view at home with the family. Go to the FEMA for Kids website (www.fema.gov/kids) for a fun and colorful way to address disasters with kids.

Fire Safety and Prevention

Prepare for a fire by stocking and training to use ABC fire extinguishers. Check your local hardware store for fire extinguishers. Each letter stands for a different type of fire. The following description of fire extinguishers types and their use is from the U.S. Fire Administration website (www.usfa.dhs.gov):

Class A extinguishers put out fires on ordinary combustible materials such as cloth, wood, rubber, paper, and many plastics.

Class B extinguishers are used on fires involving flammable liquids, such as grease, gasoline, oil, and oil-based paints.

Class C extinguishers are suitable for use on fires involving appliances, tools, or other equipment that is electrically energized or plugged in.

Class D extinguishers are designed for use on flammable metals and are often specific for the type of metal in question. These are typically found only in factories working with these metals.

Class K fire extinguishers are intended for use on fires that involve vegetable oils, animal oils, or fats in cooking appliances. These extinguishers are generally found in commercial kitchens, such as those found in restaurants, cafeterias, and with caterers. However, recently, Class K extinguishers are finding their way into the residential market for kitchen use.

There are also multi-purpose fire extinguishers such as those labeled "B-C" or "A-B-C" that can be used on two or more of the above type fires. Regardless of the type of extinguisher, place it in an area where it will be readily available, such as the kitchen, basement, and with emergency supplies on each level of the house. Put small extinguishers in cars, trucks, RVs, and boats. Have each qualified, responsible household and family member learn how to use the ABC fire extinguisher; and test them every six months, replacing as necessary.

Fighting Fires

Fires can occur anywhere, and at any time. Fires can be secondary disasters started by earthquakes and explosions and they can occur as seasonal wildfires too. Sometimes escaping and calling 9-1-1 is the best solution. If a big disaster like an earthquake causes a fire to break out, firefighters may be unable to come to the rescue right away. Prepare to be self-sufficient and learn the methods for putting out fires. The ABC extinguisher will work to put out all fires, but other methods can also be employed. Putting out a fire is simply depriving it of its fuel—air or heat. Below are some of the other ways to extinguish a fire:

- ✓ The heat of wood, cloth, and paper fires can be cooled and stopped with water.
- ✓ A towel or blanket can be used to beat out and smother a small fire.
- ✓ Grease, oil, and gas fires must be smothered. They can't be put out with water, but an ABC fire extinguisher will work.

- ✓ Ordinary kitchen items can be used to fight grease fires. A breadboard or a pan lid can be handy and accessible tools.
- ✓ Standard pantry items like baking soda, salt, and flour can be thrown on a fire to smother it.
- ✓ Sand and dirt thrown on the fire will also work to cut off oxygen and snuff out flames.
- ✓ In case of an electrical fire, do not use water. Shut off the electricity or unplug the appliance first and use the ABC extinguisher or call 9-1-1.
- ✓ If a natural gas fire breaks out, shut off the gas and use sand, dirt, or an ABC extinguisher to put it out.

Any fire that can't be controlled quickly will have to be put out by the fire department. Leave immediately, go a safe distance from the house, and call 9-1-1.

Smoke Alarms

An essential fire safety device is the battery-powered smoke alarm. These warning systems are inexpensive and easy to install, and are required by the fire marshal. Smoke alarms should be installed in sleeping areas, close to or inside bedrooms, and in hallways. A smoke alarm should be at the head of each stairway, on every floor of the house. Ten-year lithium, battery powered units are currently available at most places where batteries are sold including Lowes Hardware Stores and can be purchased for $6.00 to $19.00. They can be installed by the homeowner or an electrician can hardwire them. The devices can also be connected to a home security system and monitored by the security company. Be sure to check all smoke alarm batteries at least twice a year. You can also check with the local fire department to get the latest information and advice on fire detection systems.

General Fire Safety

Establish daily safety rules that can save lives, such as:
- ❏ Deter children from playing with matches by removing temptation. Put matches and lighters in secure, out of reach locations.
- ❏ Be aware that smoking in bed is dangerous and a common cause of fires.
- ❏ Annually inspect your electrical box, update as needed.
- ❏ Keep the number to the fire department on the emergency list and tape it to every phone.
- ❏ Watch the video prepared by the Home Safety Council on its website (www.homesafetycouncil.org) to see how safe your home is in the event of a fire. This non-profit site is dedicated to preventing home-related injuries and talks extensively about fire hazards and their causes from heaters, matches, cooking and grilling, and storage of combustible materials.

Correcting Fire Hazards

Develop the ability to spot fire hazards and correct them:
- ❏ If a window is near the kitchen stove, remove cloth curtains that could catch fire from brushing against burners.
- ❏ Never use lighter fluid or a charcoal lighter to restart or freshen up a fire, indoors or outdoors.
- ❏ Check the fireplace screen for any gaps that could allow sparks to fly out.
- ❏ While walking through the house, inspect electrical outlets for wear or overloading and replace as necessary.
- ❏ Check lamp cords, extension cords and plugs; replace worn or frayed parts.
- ❏ Move electrical cords from under rugs and avoid using nails to secure them.

- Contain solvents and gasoline in tight metal cans. Store in garages and sheds.
- Keep garbage and waste paper in closed cans outside the house.

Maintenance and Cleanup

Fires can be prevented with regular maintenance and basic cleanup:
- Have chimney professionally cleaned annually to remove flammable creosote.
- Keep all appliances clean and in good repair.
- Patrol the house to remove any rubbish, old newspapers or accumulated cardboard from closets, the basement, garage, and/or attic.
- Control grass, brush, and weeds by mowing often and keeping them low to the ground, well below knee height.
- Keep shrubbery well watered and pruned back away from the house.
- Prevent fire from leaping from landscaping to your home by taking the following actions:
  - Remove dead tree limbs and shrubs
  - Plant trees 30 feet from the house
  - Plant shrubs 20 feet from the house
  - Maintain 15–20 feet of separation between shrubs
- Find fire-resistant plants for your climate and geographic location through local nurseries. Check online (www.usfa.dhs.gov/citizens/home_fire_prev/rural).

Fire Drills

Regular fire drills are essential because they prepare you for this emergency. Be sure to time your escape as you conduct the drills, and plan at least two escape routes from every room. Statistics show that most fire fatalities occur at night when people are sleeping. According to Judy Comoletti, National Fire Protection Association (NFPA) assistant vice president for public education, eight out of 10 fire deaths occur in the home. Ms. Comoletti strongly suggests that parents find out what fire safety procedures are in place anywhere a child plans to spend a night away from home. You can view her comments at the NFPA site (http://www.sparky.org/simpson_hunt/hazards_5.html). Also, download a free sleepover checklist (www.nfpa.org).

As part of your fire safety plan, discuss what can be done if a fire breaks out at night while everyone is sleeping. Be aware that fires can spread throughout an entire room in less than three minutes. Include housekeepers or babysitters in practice fire drills. Remember, in your absence, they will be responsible for your children's care and safety. Walk through the fire drill procedures, location of supplies, emergency numbers, and escape techniques. Recent television news featured a story on an eight-year-old girl who saved herself and her five–year-old sister from a house fire by crawling out onto the roof from her second story window where the two were rescued. The girl had practiced fire drills with her parents and she knew the quick action to take when she saw smoke under the bedroom door and smelled fire.

Children will need this training, and when they have it the results are life saving. However, if they are not shown what to do, a child may react by hiding under their bed or in a closet—two actions that could prove dangerous or in the worst case, fatal. Plan several escape routes with first and second choice exit options. In short, think of every possible escape option and plan a route for that. This ensures your optimal safety. Fire drills begin with simple steps that are repeated again and again. Safety habits can be cultivated so that they eventually become second nature.

Closed Bedroom Doors

It is advisable to sleep with your bedroom door closed. If a fire starts, this helps prevent the accumulation of smoke in each room. Closed doors also set up a barrier to flames. If a smoke alarm sounds, feel the door with the back of your hand before opening it. If the door feels hot, keep it closed. Be aware that closed doors and windows can slow the rapid spread of a fire by limiting the oxygen that fuels it.

Fire Exits

As mentioned, designate two possible escape routes from each room. When in the midst of a fire, it's best to choose the most viable option and then leave quickly. The importance of getting out right away and staying out cannot be overstated. Taking time to dress or round up pets or possessions is not an option. When developing your fire exit plan and taking your household or family through the preparedness plan, keep in mind the short amount of time available during an actual fire. Also, be sure to have everyone practice escaping from their bedrooms. Doing these exercises creates a mental picture of the correct actions to take so that they kick in automatically during a crisis.

Outside Meeting Place

Plan where to meet outside of the house. Whether you choose the big oak tree or the old fence, make the spot a safe distance from the house. A safe distance is away from the heat of the fire and out of the way of responders. To judge if you're far enough away from a fire, hold your hand up and block out the fire with your thumb.

In the best-case scenario, everyone would walk to the meeting place together. If not, then even if there are two people at the meeting place, one can go call for help and one

General Preparation 55

can stay to perform the headcount and inform others that help is on the way. Do not go back into the house for possessions or rescue missions. Wait for the fire and rescue service to arrive, and report missing or trapped persons. Do not try to rescue trapped people or animals on your own. It could cost you your life.

Emergency Supplies

Emergency supplies should be kept on hand in numerous rooms, especially in bedrooms. A small emergency kit should be stored under each person's bed. Other accessible storage space can be found in closets, bookshelves, or window seats. Stored items in the kit should include towels and water in plastic jugs. Also, consider adding a pillowcase to serve several purposes. It can be wetted and put over one's head for protection or used as a mask over the nose and mouth to avoid heat and smoke. It can also be used later to tear into strips for bandaging or work as a sling. Ladders are essential for escape from a second or third story home; either a rope ladder or a tall, straight ladder can be used.

Escape Techniques

Practicing the escape plan actions regularly will allow them to become automatic. To escape from a fire, pull the towel and jug of water out from under the bed or closet. Wet the towel and roll it up to stuff in the crack under the door. This technique will keep the smoke and flames away while you escape through another exit such as a window. If the room is on the second story, pull the rope, chain or straight ladder out from storage. Secure it and climb down carefully to escape. Rope ladders can be purchased at Wal-Mart stores and online (www.walmart.com). Expect to pay between $59.00 and $89.99 for a fire escape rope ladder.

Another essential fire escape practice is the technique of crawling low on the floor to avoid smoke inhalation. The smoke from a fire is a danger in itself and many people are suffocated in fires this way every year. Smoke, toxic fumes, and heat all rise in a fire, and staying low to the ground helps you avoid all of it. Taking short breaths or covering your mouth with a towel or wet cloth will also help.

The Red Cross's "stop, drop, and roll" is an excellent method to use in teaching household members what to do if their clothing or hair catches on fire. Learning not to panic is a big part of the exercise. Stop in your tracks, drop down to the ground immediately, and smother the fire by rolling over and over, flat on the floor. This will put out the flames and extinguish the fire. Avoid instinctively running away, because the action will stir up the air, fan the flames, and feed the fire with more oxygen. Also, check online (www.childcareaware.org) for practices beyond the standard stop, drop, and roll.

Fire Safety in a Hotel or Motel

If staying at a hotel or motel, ask questions about the fire sprinkler system, smoke detectors, and evacuation plans when calling for reservations. Some hotels now offer travel safety kits to their guests and train their employees in emergency preparedness. Ask about the kits and plans in advance. On arrival, check outside the hotel grounds or a nearby street for a safe place to escape to in case of a fire. If traveling with others, plan where to meet if separated. Make sure that it's a safe distance away.

Locate the exits and stairwells inside the hotel. Be aware that if a fire starts, it is not safe to use the elevator. You will have to choose a stairwell instead. Inside the room, check for two good exits. On upper floors, make sure windows open

General Preparation 57

easily and that fire escapes or ladders are in place. Follow the same general fire safety plan for your home by sleeping with your bedroom doors closed. If you hear a smoke alarm go off, feel exit doors for heat before opening. Put a towel, flashlight, and a bottle of water under or near the bed, and have clothing ready to put on in case a quick exit is needed.

If a fire starts, use the escape techniques, like crawling low on the floor to avoid smoke, rehearsed at home. Act quickly when you first smell or see smoke or hear a fire alarm, grab the hotel key, and leave through a safe exit. Report the fire by calling 9-1-1 from a safe distance outside. You will be able to apply many of the same fire safety techniques you practiced at home for a fire emergency away from home.

Fire Safety Summary

Rehearsals and practice are a crucial part of any fire safety and emergency training. Regular fire drills are recommended by the Red Cross and by fire departments. To prepare everyone to react quickly and to escape danger, do the following:

- ❑ Buy, and learn to use and test ABC fire extinguishers.
- ❑ Learn about the various types of fires, and their dos and don'ts.
- ❑ Install smoke alarms; check batteries often.
- ❑ Sleep with bedroom doors closed.
- ❑ Do not smoke in bed.
- ❑ Keep matches away from children.
- ❑ Use correct fuses in fuse boxes.
- ❑ Do not squirt lighter fluid on barbeques or in fireplaces.
- ❑ Fix frayed lamp cords.
- ❑ Replace worn electrical outlets and sockets.
- ❑ Clean chimneys annually.
- ❑ Cleanup garages and attics.
- ❑ Store gasoline in tight cans.

- ☐ Keep trash cans outside.
- ☐ Clean and repair appliances.
- ☐ Trim grass and weeds, and cut shrubs back.
- ☐ Plan exit strategy and outside meeting spot.
- ☐ Walk escape routes together.
- ☐ Store towel, water, rope ladder, and extra clothes under bed.
- ☐ Feel doors before opening.
- ☐ Put damp towel under door crack to block smoke.
- ☐ Crawl low on the floor.
- ☐ If on fire, stop, drop, and roll to smother fire.
- ☐ Leave by pre-planned exit.
- ☐ Conduct regular fire drills.
- ☐ Use the same fire safety skills when staying in hotels and motels.

Utilities

Essential utility services of electricity, water, sewer, and gas flow to homes, businesses, and civic facilities every hour of every day; and sudden power surges, tripped circuit breakers, or blown fuses can cause temporary interruptions and inconvenience. Powerful seasonal storms deliver longer duration blackouts with greater disruption. A blizzard's ice, a thunderstorm's lightning, a hurricane's gale, and a tornado's whirlwinds have all downed power lines or snapped water, sewer, and gas supply lines. Other natural forces have proven to be catalysts of destruction and wiped out utilities too. The rumbling and reeling of an earthquake or a landslide can shake loose supply lines in its wide wake and spawn a tsunami wave or a volcanic eruption for an encore blow. Human error, mechanical failure, or cyber sabotage could bring on an equally costly disaster by shutting down a nuclear power plant and cutting off lights, heat, and water to large regions and populations.

These outages could happen any time, and it is important to prepare in advance so as to have a quick and effective emergency response. The first step in managing any disruption of utility services is locating your electrical power panel, fuse box, water main, and gas meter; and the next step is learning how to reset tripped breakers, replace fuses, and shut off power, water, or gas when necessary. Turning the water off will stave off contamination from a broken sewer line, and shutting the gas off is necessary if you smell the sulfur odor of a gas leak. Consider installing a seismic shutoff valve on the gas meter and be sure to keep shutoff wrenches nearby for easy access. Flipping breakers and electrical switches can be done by you at your electrical box, but if you shut off the gas it can only be turned back on by the gas company. It could take hours or even days for a service technician to reach and restore your gas service.

Household Utilities

During the household meeting, walk around the house together and inspect the utilities and appliances that may be damaged or need shutting off after a disaster. Rehearse quickly locating and using all the tools needed to shut off power, water, and gas. Make access quick and easy by storing the tools right next to the water main and gas meter or by the furnace. Spare shutoff tools can be kept in the emergency kit or with neighbors. Spare flashlights, batteries, and fuses should be kept in a dry place next to the electrical boxes.

Water, Electric, and Gas Shutoffs

Water Shutoff Valves
Know the location of the shutoff water valves inside your home, and practice turning them off. You can purchase a shutoff valve tool online (www.amazon.com). Be sure to read

reviews by users. Expect to pay $6.99 and up online or at your local hardware store.

To turn off a water valve on your own:
- Locate the water main on the street.
- Grab a pry bar or crowbar to dislodge the heavy metal lid that covers the water main.
- Once the lid is up, use the special water valve tool or a wrench.
- Turn the valve as far as it will turn to the right, clockwise.
- Shut the valve off and on to get familiar with each action.
- If the main valve freezes up and won't move, call the water company to service it for free. This is the company's maintenance responsibility.
- Place the pry bar and the water shutoff tool with emergency supplies or as close to the main as is convenient.

Circuit Breaker and Fuse Boxes

Know where your circuit breaker or fuse box is located and get household members to help check that all circuits are working and correctly labeled. You will also want to:
- Learn how to turn the main power off by flipping the circuit breaker switches to the "off" position.
- Replace bad fuses with the correct size fuses.
- Be sure to stock spare fuses to use in case of power outages and check on upgrading to circuit breaker boxes.
- Check electrical panels and evaluate increases in usage that could cause overloads and require upgrading of electrical panels.

Hazards can also turn up in a utilities inspection. If anything in the fuse box or breaker box appears to be loose or sparking, or if power outages or surges are occurring, call your local electric provider for an inspection. You can also call the utility company with general or troubleshooting questions and request an inspection as a safety precaution. If advised to repair or upgrade, get a written estimate from a licensed electrician. At the time of the inspection or installation, be sure to get hands-on instructions on maintaining and troubleshooting the electrical system.

Gas Meter and Shutoff Valve
You'll also want to know the location of the gas shutoff valve and shutoff tool, and periodically have your gas company check it to make sure it operates without getting stuck. Learn how to shut off all utilities (www.fema.gov/plan/prepare/utilityplan.shtm). In earthquakes, windstorms, or flooding, it is important to know how to shut off the valve at the meter in case you smell sulfur or hear the hiss of gas leaking. Gas is odorless, but gas companies add a rotten egg smell to make a leak detectable by smell. To shut off the gas, turn the valve a quarter turn clockwise. Once the gas is off, do not attempt to turn the gas back on. Call the local gas company to send a technician to re-light the pilot and restore the gas service. Because only the gas company can turn your gas back on, be prepared to be without service for hours or even days if you shut it off.

Interior and Exterior Inspection
Walk through your home to produce a punch list of jobs that need to be done. Check the Squidoo website for a list of home hazards and go through the online home hazard checklist (http://www.squidoo.com/home-hazards-and-survival-#module149744887). The inspection may reveal hazards such as precarious tree limbs that could fall on the house. A wall

with loose blocks, bricks, or mortar may require reinforcement. A garage full of hazardous and toxic materials may need to be cleaned up and reorganized for safe storage. Closet or pantry shelves with heavy items on top will have to be rearranged to lower shelves. This will minimize the risk of being struck by hurtling and potentially dangerous objects.

Decreasing Damage and Injury

A disaster can unleash dramatic and far-reaching damages. The structure of the house may be compromised from the foundation up, causing floors to slide apart, porches to separate, and garages to collapse. A chimney could fall and break through the roof. Reviewing your home's hazardous areas and eliminating concerns before a disaster strikes will limit injuries and damage on your property. Read the online guide (http://www.fdem-mediacenter.org/PDF/Emergency_Preparedness_Checklist.pdf).

Applying Safety Film

Danger also exists inside the house, from shattered windows and mirrors, flying pots and pans, runaway appliances, and toppling furniture. Applying safety film to glass in windows, skylights, mirrors, and doors will not keep the glass from shattering, but it will hold it in place in the frame. The commercial security industry has grades of safety film that can withstand the force of a hurtling boulder and a bomb explosion. Standard safety film can be purchased through a reputable window dealer and should ideally be installed by a professional. You can expect to pay a contractor for up to a full day of work, depending on how many windows you want covered. You can take the project on and do it yourself by checking with an online dealer specializing in this market (http://www.diywindowsecurity.com).

Bolting and Bracing

Many household furnishings can be well secured. Inexpensive and easy ways to secure items inside your home include: bolting down heavy furniture, attaching bookshelves to wall studs, putting safety latches on cupboard doors, bracing refrigerators, strapping down hot water heaters, installing flexible hoses on gas appliances, and eliminating anything that could fall from above beds. Check out this online list of suggestions for eliminating potential hazards via bolting and bracing (http://earthquake-preparedness.net).

Earthquake Drills

In the United States, 39 of the 50 states are earthquake prone. The Federal government has a website (www.ready.gov) to help citizens learn how to prepare their households, families, neighborhoods, communities, and states for a disaster. Earthquake drills are now practiced once a year in many states. Residents prepare all year by gathering emergency supplies and enacting neighborhood plans on a specific date and time. Over six million people took part in the 2010 California earthquake drill alone. Earthquake drills have proven effective. In Japan, regular drills have been part of citizen's lives and increased survival rates in disasters many times; most recently during the 9.0 magnitude earthquake in 2011.

Earthquake preparedness covers a broad spectrum of disaster basics, and it is therefore something that all households should implement and practice regularly. This seismic event is one we can plan for well in advance. Potential damages from earthquakes multiply with secondary disasters. Landslides, tsunamis, flooding, volcanic eruptions, gas explosions, fires, and power outages can all be triggered by earthquakes.

Personal Space and Bracing Techniques

Structural stability will be greater at the core of the house and it is important to create stability when things around you are moving. Below are some guidelines and resources for bracing yourself during a disaster. Pick an interior hallway or other safe place to get away from flying glass, falling objects, and heavy furniture.

- Try the bracing technique of sitting flat on the floor in a hallway and pressing your back against a wall while pushing your legs against the opposite wall. This leaves your arms free to help shield your head. In the past, we were told to get inside a doorway and hang on, but updated findings from the Red Cross and FEMA no longer advise that technique (http://www.earthquakecountry.info/dropcoverholdon/#notrecommended).
- You want to make yourself as small of a target as possible. See the public awareness site from The University of Memphis Center for Earthquake Research and Information about the controversy, myths, and folklore surrounding the often recommended Triangle of Life. You can also visit the U.S. Geological Survey page (http://earthquake.usgs.gov/learn/faq) for details on what to do and what not to do in a disaster.

Duck, Cover, and Hold On Tight

If shaking occurs while you're in an office, kitchen, classroom, or a bedroom, practice the Red Cross "duck, cover, and hold on tight" technique by getting under a heavy table, desk, or bed. See the Red Cross website (www.redcross.org) for more details. This type of approach provides both protection and an air space that may be needed if a ceiling collapses. Hang on tight to the furniture and move with it until the shaking stops. These techniques apply to sheltering in homes, public buildings, schools, and offices. If you're in a car, stop in a safe spot and cover your head, but remain in your car until it is safe to move about.

Exterior Hazards

Threatening Trees

Trees can stabilize slopes and soils with their root systems and their umbrellas of foliage, but they can pose hazards too. While walking around your property, make sure tree limbs are not too close to power lines leading to the house or outer buildings. In a heavy windstorm, encroaching tree limbs could crash into power lines, short them out, and spark a fire. Because of the potential damage, any threatening limbs should be pruned. Call your local power company if your power lines are affected by falling limbs. Trees that are on city property are usually maintained by the city. You may need expert advice and service from a landscape contractor, but be aware that hiring any contractor merits checking their licensing, insurance, and recent references. Another option is to work with a professional arborist. Arborists are licensed tree specialists who can evaluate tree hazards on your property and prune or remove any problem trees.

The removal of a large tree may be necessary, not to mention worth the cost, if removal keeps the tree from tumbling on top of your house during a disaster. If you are on top of or below a very steep slope, a consultation with a civil or geological engineer may be advisable. Other options include replacement of diseased trees with healthy specimens or replanting steep slopes and unstable areas with trees that have longer tap root systems. Assessing the danger and taking action in advance will protect the property, the house, and everyone living in it.

Chimneys and Power Lines

Chimneys pose a potential threat to property in the event of a disaster. The taller and heavier a chimney is, the harder it will fall. The higher off the roofline the chimney is positioned, the greater the force with which it will collapse. Chimney bricks could break through the roof and also damage the inside of the house. To protect the interior, bracing ceiling joists under the chimney with plywood may be advisable. Most building codes require external bracing to stabilize chimneys. Consider obtaining bids from licensed, bonded contractors to find out if your chimney meets required code before taking any action. This is especially advisable in seismically sensitive areas where earthquakes can strike.

Chimneys can pose fire hazards as well. Be sure to have your chimney cleaned at least once a year to greatly reduce the danger of a flue fire. Fires can also be caused by sparking and fallen power lines. While in the yard, check the location of power lines that may fall during a big storm or a disaster. Alert your neighbors of these potential dangers so that these areas can be avoided later.

Structural Hazards and Supports

The wood frame house is the most common type of housing structure. The building industry considers these structures safe and flexible. The key in keeping the house intact in a disaster, such as during an earthquake, is to make sure the house behaves as one unit. The wood frame house is designed and built to tolerate motion by flexing. The aim is to distribute force and stress evenly throughout the structure. When the house gives, its integrity is maintained and the supports

General Preparation 67

and their connections remain unbroken. In earthquake country, meeting the bracing requirements of seismic codes will help protect older wood homes. Other volatile disasters can be destructive too, and one of the greatest causes of damage to wood homes is from high winds, according to the American Society of Civil Engineers (www.asce.org). The homeowner or a contractor can easily remedy the problem through proper tie-downs to the roof. Learn more online (http://www.foremost.com/safety/home-safety/how-to-install-tie-downs-and-anchors.asp).

Foundation Bolting
Before 1950 in the United States, foundation bolting was not required by the building code. If your house was built after 1950, codes required that the frame be bolted to the foundation. If your home was built before 1950, check the United States Housing and Urban Development website (www.hud/gov/office/lead/LBPguide.pdf) for booklets on renovating homes with lead based paint. To ensure the safety and stability of any house, make sure the foundation and frame are bolted together. To get started, contact several licensed contractors or seismic retrofitters. Referrals for qualified contractors may be available through homebuilder's associations and local construction contractor boards.

Hiring a Contractor
There are several smart tactics you can employ when hiring a contractor that will make the project and your life a lot easier:
- ❏ Check out a contractor before you sign a contract by first calling the contractor's board to verify the status of his license.
- ❏ Research any documented complaints and open claims.

- Check the history and reliability of the contractor to ensure the work will be done timely and up to professional standards.
- Get insurance information with the dollar limits on liability coverage and the type of bond and its dollar limit. Make sure the coverage is adequate for your project.
- Ask for three recent references and be sure to follow-up on them.
- Always get a written bid in advance of any work detailing project costs, deposits, schedules, timelines, and change orders.
- Ask how much expediting, trip, and shopping charges will run.
- A good rule of thumb in choosing a contractor is to get three bids and take the one in the middle.
- Both parties will sign the bid and convert it into a legal contract. Be sure to get a copy with the total cost of the project that was agreed upon.
- For clarity, have the labor costs and material costs spelled out separately. Find out what the markup is on parts and materials. For a breakdown on how to ask for a contractor's bid and how to evaluate a bid, check online (http://homerepair.about.com/od/workingwithcontractors1/a/tu_how2_bid.htm).
- Be sure to specify in writing that the work must be done to a workmanlike standard, the industry's term for quality work.
- Allow for delays and remedies in the contract because they will happen.
- Spell everything out as much as possible to ensure that the job is done to your specifications.
- Additions in labor, upgrades in materials, or any job

General Preparation

modifications need a Change Order form that both parties must sign off on.
- Check online (http://homerepair.about.com/od/workingwithcontractors1/a/tu_how2_bid.htm) for what change orders are, when you need them, and additional costs to expect.

Once the contract is signed with the specifications laid out, use it to monitor the progress of the project. At the end of the job, conduct a walk through with the contractor and make a punch list of things to be completed or redone. Sign off on the job only when all the work on the punch list is performed and the project is completed to satisfaction. Only then should the contractor receive final payment.

Retrofitting By Owner

While this is not an easy job, experts say that it *can* be done by the homeowner. It is estimated that those who retrofit their own homes can spend a third of what a contractor charges. Even if you hire a contractor, industry experts recommend taking a class on retrofitting so that you know what is being done. Check the videos online at Earthquake Tech (www.earthquaketech.com) that walk you through a retrofit.

Saving money can be a big plus when handling the retrofitting yourself. But, before taking on the project, educate yourself on what the job entails in time, labor, and materials and tools. Go online to see what is offered to homeowners who want to retrofit their own homes (http://www.seattle.gov/dpd/Emergency/Earthquakes/Home_Retrofit_Program/DPDS_005871.asp). While this was created for the Seattle community, it will give you a good idea of what is necessary for a home retrofitting project anywhere.

Bolting floor joists directly to the foundation of the house is hard, physically demanding work. It is done in small crawl spaces wielding heavy, hand-held power tools and wearing cumbersome protective equipment. Weigh the risks of injury before taking the job on. Be sure to apply for any required building permits before beginning the work. The cost of retrofitting, whether hired out or not, will be a fraction of the cost of catastrophic damage to an unsecured dwelling.

Sheathing

In the 1989 San Francisco World Series quake, many structures that failed to hold up and collapsed in on themselves were of the "soft story" type. Soft story refers to buildings of wood frame construction with large openings at the bottom, like parking garages. An excellent article (http://www.cityofalamedaca.gov/City-Hall/Soft-Story-Buildings) describes the building failures in California after the 1989 earthquake. Garage walls and ceilings can be sheathed with half-inch plywood to strengthen the structure to avoid what happened in the California quake. To meet seismic code, structural reinforcement, sheathing, or bracing should be done in any area where remodeling has occurred, and around picture windows. For professional advice, call a licensed structural engineer to determine the adequacy of existing plywood siding in your home. Current building and seismic codes will have to be met and permits must be posted to move forward with the work.

Bolting

Check your county agency website for online retrofit handbooks for the do-it-yourself home repair types. A visit to your local building supply dealer will also prove educational along with visiting the National Hurricane Center website (www.nhc.noaa.gov). Choose the tab "Be Prepared" followed

General Preparation 71

by "Securing Your Home" to locate the section on retrofitting. Hurricanes are the strongest windstorms and do the most damage, so retrofitting to these standards will provide you with the greatest protection. Detailed descriptions of the materials needed to retrofit your home are also provided.

A sizeable array of metal connectors are available to secure any joint in the house. Your local hardware store is a good resource for questions on the hardware that pertains to your geographic area. When you have the right brackets, you can securely anchor porches and decks to the main house. You can also secure plumbing and gas lines every few feet with straps connected to walls, ceilings, or floor joists.

Interior Hazards

Use the following room inventory to identify the danger points of each room in your home. From there, secure items that could be hazardous or cause injury and damage. Be sure to pick a safe place in every room for household members to be in when disaster strikes.

Living Room

The living room is where company is received on special occasions. It is the most formal room in the house. Collectibles, art, mirrors, and antiques are often displayed here. Tall and heavy furniture such as armoires, entertainment cabinets, trunks, sofas, grandfather clocks, and bookcases are often used to furnish the living room. Safeguard your valuables, secure hazards, and bolt down the top-heavy items. Following is a list of steps to take in securing the living room:

- ❑ Secure pictures: close hooks, screw frames to wall studs.
- ❑ Safety-film skylights, windows, sliders, and French doors.
- ❑ Secure and safety-film mirrors.

- ❏ Secure artwork: close hooks, screw frames to wall studs.
- ❏ Bracket bookshelves to wall studs.
- ❏ Bracket TV, VCR/DVD, and stereo or strap together with Velcro.
- ❏ Bolt large furniture to wall studs or to the floor.
- ❏ Weight vases, ceramics, and sculptures with beanbags.
- ❏ Use putty-fastener to secure collectibles to shelves.
- ❏ Move heavy items to lower shelves.

Kitchen

This can sometimes be the most dangerous room in the house. China, glassware, and pots and pans may fly missile-like out of cabinets and shelves in the event of a disaster. The refrigerator and stove may spring free and bulldoze anything in its path. Exploding gas appliances can torch the house and injure its occupants. Have a healthy respect for these hazards and stay away from the kitchen in any disaster. Following is a list of steps to take in making the kitchen safer and more secure:

- ❏ Brace the refrigerator and keep heavy objects off the top of it.
- ❏ Use safety-film on skylights, windows, sliders, and French doors.
- ❏ Secure the dishwasher.
- ❏ Install non-skid padding on shelves.
- ❏ Install child-security drawer and cabinet guards.
- ❏ Protect plates, bowls, and cups with foam sleeves.
- ❏ Protect glasses and wine bottles in foam containers or compartments with cardboard dividers, such as wine cases.
- ❏ Pack heirloom china, crystal, and other valuables in newspaper. Then, place in boxes and store in a secure place.
- ❏ Install flex hose on gas appliances.

General Preparation 73

Bonus Room

This is often a multipurpose room with heavy traffic. The household and family gather here on a daily basis. Beware of all glass in the room and tall, heavy furniture, such as entertainment centers and bookshelves. All large and heavy pieces should be secured. Following is a list of steps to take in making the bonus room safer:

- ☐ Move heavy objects to lower shelves.
- ☐ Secure pictures: close hooks, screw frames to wall studs.
- ☐ Apply safety film to glass, skylights, and sliders.
- ☐ Secure artwork and photographs using putty (available at art stores).
- ☐ Bracket bookshelves to wall studs.
- ☐ Anchor entertainment center to wall studs.
- ☐ Bracket TV, VCR/DVD, stereo or stick together with Velcro.
- ☐ Bolt large furniture to the floor.
- ☐ Weight vases, ceramics, and sculptures with beanbags.
- ☐ Fasten collectibles to shelves (use putty available at art stores).

Dining Room

Increasingly, families live in their kitchens and bonus rooms. The dining room is often designated for more formal gatherings. Following is a list of steps to make the dining room safer and more secure:

- ☐ Inspect any chandeliers to see if they are braced from the attic. Secure them as needed, by yourself or through a contractor.
- ☐ Secure mirrors: close hooks, screw frame to wall studs.
- ☐ Bracket side tables, buffets, hutches.
- ☐ Remove casters from any large pieces of furniture, tables.

- Install non-skid padding where serving dishes, silver, and crystal are kept.
- Install child-security drawer and cabinet guards.
- Use putty-fastener for vases and candlesticks.
- Anchor buffet, highboy, hutches, and side tables to wall studs.
- Have a professional window contractor apply safety-film on large glass and picture windows.
- Move heavy objects to lower shelves.

Bathroom

Bathrooms are often filled with mirrors, windows, skylights, shower doors, and glass containers of all kinds. To avoid cuts from broken glass, use unbreakable plastic containers as much as possible. If cleaning supplies are kept in the bathroom, chemical spills may have to be contended with in a disaster. If possible, limit the number of toxic substances stored in the bathroom, or use earth-friendly cleaning products. Following is a list of steps to make the bathroom safer:

- Secure hanging plants.
- Apply safety-film on glass, mirrors, windows, and skylights.
- Install child-security drawer and cabinet guards.
- Secure pictures, close hooks, screw frames to wall studs.
- Store shampoos, razors, and breakables in drawers.
- Eliminate glass containers and replace them with non-breakable plastic containers.
- Move heavy objects to lower shelves.

Bedroom

The bedroom is your place of rest. First and foremost, eliminate hazards like framed art and mirrors that could fall from

General Preparation

over the bed and cause injury. Remove any tapestries, wall hangings or weavings from above the bed so they won't drop down on anyone sleeping there. Stabilize the bed with carpeting, remove casters, or brace legs with wooden blocks to prevent the bed from moving. Also, secure or eliminate heavy furniture. As discussed previously, be sure to designate two exits from every bedroom and walk the escape route beforehand so everyone is familiar with it. Following is a list of steps to make the bedroom safer and more secure:

- ❏ Secure pictures: close hooks and screw frames to wall studs.
- ❏ Secure mirrors by bolting and use safety film on the glass as a protective coating.
- ❏ Have a contractor apply safety-film on large windows and skylights.
- ❏ Draw drapes or Venetian blinds overnight.
- ❏ Bolt dressers, armoires, and desks to wall studs.
- ❏ Install child security drawers and cabinet guards.
- ❏ Remove heavy items and mirrors from above beds.
- ❏ Remove wall tapestries and weavings from over beds.
- ❏ Remove casters from beds or block legs.
- ❏ Attach bunk beds, bracket to wall studs.
- ❏ Bracket TV, VCR/DVD, stereo or fasten with Velcro.
- ❏ Bracket bookshelves to each other or to wall studs.
- ❏ Move heavy objects to lower shelves and not above the bed.

Office or Den

The office or den is a catchall room for the whole family. Its functions include reading, working on the computer, watching television, talking on the telephone, and listening to music. Following is a list of steps to making this room safer:

- ☐ Remove rollers or casters from furniture.
- ☐ Bracket bookshelves to wall studs.
- ☐ Secure file cabinet drawers.
- ☐ Bracket TV, VCR/DVD, and stereo equipment.
- ☐ Secure computer, printer, and accessories.
- ☐ Store and secure computer external hard drive on the floor.
- ☐ Secure exercise equipment.
- ☐ Apply safety-film to windows, mirrors.

Garage and Laundry

The garage and laundry room receive almost as much use as the kitchen. The garage is home to tools, ladders, outdoor and athletic equipment, building supplies, generators, power mowers, gardening supplies, paint, bicycles and motorcycles, cars, and boats. The laundry room houses the washer and dryer, and it can also be used as an additional storage option. Both of these locations pose hazards and security risks. Following is a list of safe storage steps to take:

- ☐ Place firewood in heavy boxes bolted to the floor.
- ☐ Store house paint, cleaning chemicals, motor oil in a shed.
- ☐ Use child-security drawer and cabinet latches.
- ☐ Secure tools in containers that latch.
- ☐ Tie down building materials with bungee cords.
- ☐ Secure propane tanks.
- ☐ Move heavy objects to lower shelves.
- ☐ Secure refrigerator or freezer doors.
- ☐ Use flexible hoses for gas clothes dryer.
- ☐ Block washer or bolt in place.
- ☐ Secure hot water heater with plumber's tape or bolt in place.

After the Disaster Plan

Before a disaster strikes is when you want to prepare for what will happen afterwards. Delegate after-the-disaster jobs in advance, according to individual ability. Everyone can do his or her part to pitch in. Make a checklist of the jobs for each individual and post on a bulletin board or on the refrigerator so everyone in the household knows what their responsibilities will be. Knowing what to do will help each person respond quickly. Young children may be placed in charge of getting pets inside and offering them food and comfort. Older siblings can help direct and aid younger brothers and sisters.

Headcount and First Aid

After a disaster or other dramatic event, the area may be filled with broken glass, rubble, mud, and water. Before jumping into action, put on your protective clothing and heavy shoes from the under the bed kits. The first order of business will be taking a head count of all present and searching for those injured or trapped. First aid may be needed. After injuries are treated, elderly or disabled neighbors can be checked and treated.

Separation of Household and Family Members

Thinking about what could happen if household members become separated is important in the disaster discussion and planning process. Decide where to meet after a disaster, both inside the house and a safe distance from the house. Address the questions of what to do if everyone ends up in different parts of town, or stuck at work or at school, traveling by car on the freeway, at the store, in a theater, in a high rise building, or at an event or game. Exploring the different venues and thinking through actions in advance will enhance survival skills amidst the chaos, confusion, and turmoil of any disaster.

Everyone should have the out-of-area contact person's telephone number saved or written down so they can keep in touch with other household members. Use your personal cell phone to check your household plan and actions saved in your phone. Review phone applications you can use to help you before a disaster happens from our Resource Guide. Placing a house key in an outside hiding place will provide anyone returning home with ready access as well. Having an extra house key and car key in each emergency kit is recommended.

Staying or Leaving

The household leader will be in charge of directing the action. He or she will make the judgment call on whether to stay or go. If immediate evacuation is necessary, the clean-up jobs will have to wait until it is announced by authorities that it is safe to return home. Minor damage like a hole in the roof, broken windows, fallen plaster, loose bricks, and a power outage may allow for staying in the house. If damage to the structure is more severe, it may be possible to camp in the yard until repairs can be made.

Sheltering in Place

In some emergencies, it is best to hunker down and stay in the house. The Red Cross calls this action sheltering in place (www.redcross.org). Walk around together outside and inside to evaluate risks, make punch lists of repairs and clean-up, and choose a safe place to take cover during the disaster. Closets and interior hallways away from glass

General Preparation 79

and top-heavy furniture are one option for shelter. Getting underneath a table could also be a good place to duck for cover. Some households have basement areas or safe rooms designed for this purpose. If you and your household are interested in creating this type of shelter, both safe room and exterior shelter kits are currently available through disaster supply companies, or contact us for recommendations (www.naturaldisastersbook.com).

Reassuring Children

Disasters strike suddenly and frighten everyone. When chaos disrupts daily, dependable routines, children can feel especially vulnerable. Once the physical danger of the event has passed, children will need to be reassured. It is important for parents to be calm and set a good example for how to behave. Parental panic reactions and acting out will trigger the same in children. Below are important techniques to utilize when reassuring your children after a disaster strikes:

- ❑ Communicate the basics of the situation and explain what the plan is.
- ❑ Assure children that conditions are temporary and will normalize eventually.
- ❑ Emphasize that you all will be staying together and working through the transition.
- ❑ If evacuating, keep children with the rest of the household or family as much as possible while seeking assistance and housing.
- ❑ Ease children's discomfort and anxiety by encouraging them to talk about the disaster, and their feelings.
- ❑ Meet children at eye level by kneeling or squatting down to provide a safe format in which they can express their emotions.

- ❏ Tune in to their need to talk through what is troubling them by listening intently to them.
- ❏ Accept what they say, and offer sympathy and understanding to comfort them and pave the way to healthy adjustment.
- ❏ Open a dialogue so that everyone can share their feelings to aid the healing process.

In addition, you'll want to limit children's television exposure to disaster news and monitor all television watching, as regular programs can be interrupted with late breaking bulletins. Continuous television newscasts of disasters may make children think that multiple incidents have happened. Fear of continuing danger and disaster could grow and be expressed in aggressive or regressive behavior, loss of appetite, and bad dreams. Whatever their origins, fears of injury, death, and abandonment are very real for children. It is important, as a parent or caregiver, to be mindful of these fears and maintain close communication with children before, during, and after a disaster.

After Disaster Jobs

After the disaster, once the decision to stay has been made, it will be necessary to prioritize tasks. Putting out fires and checking for gas leaks should be first on the list. If gas fumes or hissing from gas connectors indicate leaks, turn off the gas service to prevent explosions or fires. Use ABC fire extinguishers, buckets of sand, or heavy blankets to smother small fires. If the fire can't be controlled, escape to a place a safe distance away and call 9-1-1. If appliances are sparking, unplug them. In case of a sewer backup, be sure to plug the tub and sink drains and shut toilet lids, and switch to portable camping toilets or buckets with tight lids. After the

General Preparation

emergency jobs are done, it will no doubt be time to eat. The person in charge of preparing and serving the family's first post-disaster meal will offer welcome respite from commotion and chaos. Serve comfort food from the pre-planned menu, and have children assist with serving and cleaning up. Bring in normalcy whenever possible, while encouraging sharing and open communication.

Children's Jobs
Assign your children jobs to allow them to pitch in on the family's recovery. As active helpers, they will feel like part of the solution and will feel a sense of normalcy. The tasks of washing the dishes, wrapping up garbage, or sweeping up debris will keep children busy and allow less time for worry. Rounding up and caring for pets, and picking up scattered items are other jobs children can perform.

Summary of After Disaster Jobs—For Children
- Find and feed pets.
- Help with clean-up.
- Assist with the first meal.
- Send emergency notifications if possible by phone or computer regarding family safety.

Summary of After Disaster Jobs—For Adults
- Put out fires.
- Render first aid.
- Check for gas leaks.
- Unplug appliances.
- Plug sink and tub drains.
- Sweep up debris and glass.
- Repair broken windows.

Water Access and Purification

Drinking water prevents dehydration, and it is necessary for survival. Set aside one gallon of water per day for each person or pet, for drinking and washing. Following a violent storm or disaster, do not drink tap water, as it may be contaminated. Purchase water purification tablets for emergencies. They can be found at local outdoor stores such as REI (www.rei.com) and cost roughly $5.00 for 50 tablets. If you do not have stored water available, there are a few other ways to harvest clean water. Water from the toilet tank may be used if no chemical treatment agent is present. The untreated tank water can be purified by boiling it for 5–10 minutes. *Note: Do not use water from the toilet bowl.* Frozen ice cubes in the refrigerator can also be used for drinking water.

Water can be harvested from the hot water heater, provided the glass liner is intact.

- ❑ Inspect the water heater carefully.
    - If any broken glass is present, do not use the water.
    - If the liner is cracked, extremely minute glass particles that are invisible to the eye may be present.
    - Drinking this water can cause internal damage if any glass particles are ingested.
    - Straining the water through a cloth is not recommended.
    - Double check the liner to make sure it is intact before getting the water out of the tank.
- ❑ First, turn off the gas or electric heat source. If the valve on the top of the tank won't open, turn on a hot water faucet inside the house. Then place a clean jug or vessel under the tap and fill it with water. Refill as necessary.

Evacuation

It is vital to be mentally and physically prepared to evacuate anytime lives are endangered. Every emergency plan should include an evacuation plan. Evacuation may be viewed as the last resort, but it is sometimes the only choice when the threat is critical. Many disasters, including hazardous chemical spills, earthquakes, tsunamis, wildfires, and terrorist attacks, will strike with little warning and require immediate evacuation. Emergency supplies stored in easy to move backpacks or garbage cans with roller wheels will allow for a quick departure. Being able to carry some possessions and supplies will enhance self-sufficiency and sustainability. This is particularly true if leaving on foot in a remote area where it may take days to reach another source of food or water.

Knowing When to Go

Evacuation does not always require official notification. Trust your observations; make the judgment call and escape. If a wildfire torches the tinderbox prairie below your house, it is time to run. Don't wait for the flames to whip up the hill and engulf your house. Grab the emergency kit and evacuate. After a thunderstorm's two-day deluge washes the river over its banks and onto your land, it is time to escape the flood.

Situational awareness is critical and will determine whether evacuation is appropriate. When blackened skies and whirling winds signal a tornado, go to your resources and tune to the National Weather Service news feeds, aerial images, warning messages, and mapping tools (www.weather.gov). You can also review the National Terror website (www.nationalterroralert.com/evacuation-plan) ahead of time for details on when to evacuate. Being alert to changing conditions is a big part of preparedness, and changes you observe in your physical surroundings may require a quick exit.

Disaster Warnings

Disaster warnings allow lead-time before evacuation. Hurricanes are usually preceded by small craft warnings and storm warnings. Official warnings of volcanic eruptions always forecast evacuation. By the time a volcano launches its rocket of red-hot lava up into the sky, it is time to be far away. Tsunamis are triggered by earthquakes and volcanic eruptions. Their warnings usually come in response to a reported seismic recording of an earthquake. Before the ocean wave torpedoes inland, it's time to flee to higher ground. Volcanoes can brew for a period of time before they erupt, and the sulfur fumes and plumes of smoke may be a signal to go. Knowing the warning systems and paying attention to television and online news and Emergency Alert Systems (EAS) will lay out the facts, the severity of the breaking storm or calamity, which evacuation routes to take, and where to seek shelter (www.fcc.gov). Also, install an emergency alert phone app on your mobile device.

Relocating

If authorities designate the neighborhood or larger community as unsafe, relocating away from home for more than several weeks may be necessary. Contact friends or relatives who live a safe distance away, or arrange for transitional housing for household members and pets. Mark on a local map the relocation destinations, along with at least two alternate evacuation routes, in case some are blocked. Because you may have to walk out of the area on foot, prepare by both walking and driving the routes beforehand and familiarize everyone with the escape plan. The map can be included in

General Preparation

the disaster kit along with a compass and a list of destination telephone numbers. Utilize Google maps for a resource that you can share among household members and the out-of-area emergency contact person. Save this information to your cell phone, tablet, or computer for easy access.

Emergency Shelters and Lodging

Having several destinations as shelter options will allow for some flexibility. Mark possible hotels, motels, and community emergency shelters on the map. If pets will be with you, be aware that most shelters will not accept them. Pet-friendly hotels and motels will charge a fee, and they may have restrictions on breeds, sizes, and the number of animals. Ask the local veterinarian for several names of good boarding kennels ahead of time, as reservations may be needed. Keep the lodging and kennel phone numbers with the disaster kit and pet supplies. If you have a cell phone, you can call while you're in route.

Updating Destination Information

Call from your cell phone, text, use social media, or email your out-of-area contact so he or she has your latest destination and routing information. Separated household and family members may be communicating through the out-of-area contact, so they will need to know where others are traveling or staying. Phone apps exist that can alert everyone including your out-of-area contact person to your location, making it possible to upload messages without a computer.

Red Cross Stations and Government Aid

Government aid is available in distressed areas when an official state of emergency is declared. Communities affected by a disaster will be a priority for emergency responders, paramedics, and firefighters. Utility companies will attempt to restore power and basic services. The Red Cross will set up first aid stations to treat injuries, provide medical care, and supply food, water, and shelter, but this may not happen right away.

Emergency service providers such as fire, police, and first responders will handle citywide emergencies before they handle neighborhood and individual resident needs. Typically, you want to be prepared to be on your own for the first three days to three weeks in the case of a major disaster. In the interim, being prepared and having supplies, food, and water will be necessary. Know how recovery agencies communicate in a disaster and store that information in your mobile device. Hashtags for use on Twitter are often set up within hours of a disaster to direct people to food, water, shelter, and medical care in the affected area.

Insurance Vouchers and Claims

Insurance companies may be of immediate help after a disaster. They will set up a temporary base of operations in an accessible, central location. Cash or vouchers for food, lodging, and transportation will be issued. Full insurance coverage is always the best defense against loss of property and loss of use; and it is best to have policy information and the household inventory with you in the emergency kit. Federal aid will not arrive until a disaster assessment is done and that could take days, weeks, or months. Call, text, email, or Twitter your insurance company as soon as possible to find out what aid will be available following a disaster, and be sure to ask about the relaxation of any policies in the midst of a crisis. Check for help from the non-profit insurance center online (www.uphelp.org).

General Preparation 87

Evacuation Tips

- ❏ Buy an Emergency Broadcast System radio or get a phone app that turns your phone into an emergency radio (see Resource Guide).
- ❏ Practice leaving the house in five to 30 minutes. Run through which supplies and kits to grab.
- ❏ Know where to go for shelter, and how to get there via your preplanned walking and driving routes.
- ❏ Know the location of pet kits and carriers, how to contain pets inside safely and get them ready for transport in a hurry.
- ❏ Keep pets' vaccination papers taped to carriers as pet shelters will ask for them.
- ❏ Identify and understand warning sirens, horns, or bells in your area.
- ❏ Be aware of changing weather and environmental conditions.
- ❏ Tune into television news, radio broadcasts, and warnings; and follow directions given by authorities.
- ❏ Secure the house quickly when exiting.
- ❏ Know how to call the out-of-area contact person with reports, updates on destinations, and messages.
- ❏ Call, text, email, or Twitter your contact person to relay or retrieve your insurance or medical information.

Conditions Requiring Evacuation:

- ✓ Out of control interior fire
- ✓ Encroaching wildfire
- ✓ Explosions
- ✓ Bomb Threats
- ✓ Flooding
- ✓ Asbestos leakage

- ✓ Landslide
- ✓ Unstable, shifting ground
- ✓ Collapsed buildings
- ✓ Tsunami warnings
- ✓ Typhoon warnings
- ✓ Tornado warnings
- ✓ Volcano warning
- ✓ Gas leaks
- ✓ Chemical spills
- ✓ Hazardous materials leak
- ✓ Nuclear reactor leaks
- ✓ Terrorist biological attack
- ✓ Terrorist chemical attack
- ✓ Terrorist nuclear attack or dirty bombs

Plans

Insurance Company Plan

Talking with your insurance agent about your homeowner's or renter's policy will help provide you with more information on claims reimbursement and the next steps after a disaster. Below is a list of questions to review with your insurance agent:

- ❑ In the pandemonium caused by a disaster, how and when will your insurance company respond to the claims of its policyholders?
- ❑ Will tents be erected in the middle of town, or are there other provisions for temporary operating facilities?
- ❑ Will a homeowner be given a voucher to stay in a hotel if the house is seriously damaged or destroyed? How will meals be handled?
- ❑ How much documentation or on-site investigation by

General Preparation 89

claims representatives will be necessary before disaster claims can be settled?
- ❑ What will happen if you have been forced to evacuate and don't have your insurance paperwork or policy information?
- ❑ What will happen if no household inventory, videotape, or any immediate supporting records are available?

Homeowner's and Renter's Insurance

For most homeowners, their home is their biggest asset, as well as a major investment. You will want to protect that asset and avoid an overwhelming financial burden due to a disaster. Being underinsured could mean losing all of your home equity. It could mean depleting your savings or borrowing to pay replacement costs on the house and its contents. Out of pocket costs for daily living expenses of temporary lodging and meals would deplete cash and compound the stress. Liability issues could be raised. People injured on your property could sue for damages. It is critical for many reasons to buy enough insurance. Even if you do not presently carry disaster coverage, you may find the monthly premiums affordable in the face of traumatic losses. It is best to do this research now, before disaster strikes. The top 20 Insurance Recovery Tips from United Policyholders, a national non-profit on insurance concerns, can be found online (www.unitedpolicyholders.org).

What if a catastrophic event were suddenly to befall you, your loved ones, or your property? Insurance money, not government assistance, will make the difference in rebuilding after a disaster. For this reason, good insurance coverage is a fundamental part of your disaster plan. It is both prudent and necessary to anticipate and prepare for a possible insurance claim well before a disaster happens. Be proactive now and call your insurance agent to set up a meeting to review your coverage.

Some agencies offer an alert service that you can sign up for if you live in a disaster prone area. They can email, text, or beep you regarding an impending disaster. Review your policy with your agent on a regular basis. Annual insurance audits are recommended by risk management experts, and it will help you stay current on your needs, and protect your interests. Find out from your agent if your current homeowner's or renter's coverage is adequate and make necessary changes.

Your insurance agent will be able to help you assess potential risks, understand liabilities, and maintain proper insurance. A policy review will also address updating coverage as necessary. Ask questions and take notes to compare costs of insurance premiums to the risks. Weigh what other assets would be put in jeopardy from damages and liability claims to make an informed decision. Always confirm oral promises of additional coverage in writing and retain current copies of your policies.

Some disasters are not covered in standard homeowner's or renter's policies. Those living on a flood plane will be required by their mortgage lenders to purchase flood insurance. The additional premium will prove well worth the monthly or annual cost if a flood hits. In earthquake-prone areas all over the world, insurance agents often advise their customers to carry earthquake insurance. This is a *Difference in Conditions* policy, commonly known as a DIC, and it carries an additional annual premium and a 10 percent to 20 percent deductible. Without this policy damages from an earthquake would not be covered. The powerful seismic

General Preparation

events can generate other earth movement disasters like landslides and volcanic eruptions and trigger fires, floods, tsunamis, gas line explosions, power plant outages, and sewer line backups. The numerous natural and man-made events that follow an earthquake multiply the damage and destruction. DIC policies like the ones that cover earthquakes are available for landslides as well. Sewer line backup protection can also be added to your policy at an additional cost.

When disasters hit, good insurance coverage can rescue the policyholder from financial catastrophe. If you do not have disaster coverage yet, the time to look into getting it is now. If a state of emergency has recently hit your community, a moratorium on insurance coverage may be issued. This will be temporary. Shop for coverage and prepare to get on the waiting list before another occurrence. The following are sample questions to help you open a dialogue with your insurance agent:

- ❏ What exactly does my homeowner's policy cover and exclude coverage on?
- ❏ What disasters does it cover?
- ❏ What disasters do I have to prepare for in this geographic location?
- ❏ In a hurricane region, am I covered for wind damage in my standard policy?
- ❏ What is the deductible?
- ❏ How is the worth of my property calculated for a claim?
- ❏ Is my claim calculated on what I owe on the house, on appraised value, or on current market value?
- ❏ Is my house insured for the full value of the mortgage? Is the land the house is built on insured?
- ❏ How much insurance should I carry to get full payment for my losses from my insurance company?

- ❑ Can I get a building ordinance rider to cover up to 50 percent of the costs of rebuilding my home should it have to be upgraded? Will this cover construction and materials costs that have increased over time? How much will the rider cost per month and per year?
- ❑ How can I prove added value for remodeling and improvements? Do I need the receipts and invoices? Will photographs be proof?
- ❑ Am I insured for replacement value of my personal property, belongings, and valuables? Are my possessions subject to depreciation? What is the cost difference?
- ❑ What is my liability coverage limit? What is the limit for medical injuries?
- ❑ Who does the liability portion cover?
- ❑ Is there a moratorium in this area on disaster insurance? And if so, when can I get on the waiting list? When will policies start being written again?
- ❑ What if my home does not meet current building code? Are some things grandfathered in, or do I need to have upgrades?
- ❑ Will I pay more in premiums for a masonry home, a home on stilts or a home built on a landfill? Will coverage be limited?
- ❑ How does the insurance company determine loss of use?
- ❑ Does a loss of use mean that my transportation and lodging costs are covered if my home is unsafe following a disaster? Does that mean I can stay in a hotel after a disaster and charge it to my insurance?
- ❑ What dollar limit, if any, is there on loss of use?
- ❑ What kind of inspection would I need to get in order to determine the structural integrity of my home?
- ❑ Does the insurance office have an engineer available to inspect structures after the disaster?

General Preparation 93

- What does the term "dwelling extensions" mean? Does it apply to my decks, fences, and unattached structures?
- What is the formula for calculating dwelling extension limits?
- How much are my shrubbery, trees, hedges, and landscaping insured for?
- In case of an earthquake, is an aftershock a separate incident? Is it all on one claim if there are several aftershocks?
- What if there are aftershocks months after the event?
- Do I need a separate policy for fine art and antiques?
- Do I need a floater policy for camera equipment, computers, jewelry, and furs?
- Will my flood insurance cover me if my house was built on a flood plain?
- What if my house is not in a flood plain but subject to flash flooding?
- Will my homeowner's policy extend to my automobile and safe deposit box? Will I be covered where I travel?
- If I am forced to evacuate, will my policy remain in place, even though the premises may be unsecured?
- What if the windows of my house were blown out by a storm and the house was robbed? How will theft claims be resolved?
- Do I need an appraisal to guarantee replacement costs on heirlooms and antiques? What does the term "garage sale" cost mean?
- Do you have an appraiser to recommend?
- Do I need a rider policy for plate glass?
- If I have disaster coverage, will it deter or make me exempt from emergency assistance after a disaster?
- Does earthquake insurance cover other earth movements, such as volcanic eruptions or landslides?

- ❏ Does earthquake insurance cover tsunamis that follow another disaster later?
- ❏ If residing on the ocean, on a lake, or on riverfront property, is it possible to obtain tsunami insurance? What is the deductible?
- ❏ Is damage done to my home by a disaster tax-deductible?
- ❏ If I suffer a property loss in a disaster and the government offers Federal assistance, can the loss be deducted on my income taxes?
- ❏ Would the loss apply to the current year or the prior year?
- ❏ Is my car covered by my homeowner's policy if it is in the garage at the time of a disaster and the garage collapses?
- ❏ Is the car covered if it is parked on the street at a friend's? Can my automobile insurance cover the damage?
- ❏ If I am traveling at the time of a disaster, is my rental car covered?
- ❏ Is damage done to my car tax-deductible if caused by a disaster?
- ❏ Is damage done to my trees or shrubbery by an earthquake, hurricane, tornado, flood, fire, or other sudden event tax-deductible?
- ❏ If my neighbor's house catches fire due to a disaster and the fire spreads to my house, am I covered on my policy or his?
- ❏ If an explosion occurs as the result of a disaster, am I covered?
- ❏ If I had to demolish my home in a disaster area or relocate, may I claim the loss?
- ❏ If my property wasn't damaged by the initial storm, but

is now in danger of landslides or mud slides from the storm, may I claim the loss if I am forced to sell?
- ❑ If authorities order evacuation, forcing me to abandon the house, can I claim a loss?
- ❑ Does my policy cover terrorist attacks?

Documentation for Insurance Claims

If you suffer a loss of personal property, you will be expected to provide proof of purchase via sales receipts or a professional appraisal and videotape, CDs, or photographs of your belongings. Insurance companies rely on this evidence to verify inventories of possessions and valuables. Documentation greatly aids in settling claims quickly. Be sure to retain all documentation for your insurance claims. You can read online more about doing your own home inventory (http://www.knowyourstuff.org/iii/login.html). There are many services offered through insurance agencies by private for-profit businesses that will videotape your possessions as a record of verification.

Sales Receipts

These verify the date and cost of your purchases. Canceled checks, credit card slips, and copies of contracts all serve as adequate proof. Copy sales receipts and store copies in the emergency kit, safe deposit box, and also send to your out-of-area contact person. Store records of purchases on removable hard drives with your emergency kit or in the cloud for easy access no matter where you may end up.

Professional Appraisals

In the event of a disaster, it is helpful to have appraisals done for valuables that you do not have receipts for, such as inherited or antique goods. This will allow your insurance claims to be processed smoothly and ensure that you are refunded for any lost items. Furs, antiques, fine art, heirloom pieces, gifts, collections, and jewelry all need to be appraised every five years or as you add pieces. Have the appraiser provide you with a written, dated inventory, and statement of value. Appraisers' charges can vary. Ask your insurance agent to recommend a reliable professional, an estate sale business, or an auction house.

Appraisals of possessions and valuables are usually done in your home. For portable items such as silver, jewelry, crystal, and china, a local jeweler or antique seller may provide you with the information and documentation you need. For silver or fine china, a fork or a serving plate can establish the pattern and allow the appraiser to accurately give a base value. Finally, keep copies of your appraisal(s) in the emergency kit, in the safe deposit box, and send to your out-of-area contact person.

Videotape

Some insurance agents will provide videotaping service to their clients by visiting them at home and making a tape of possessions and valuables at little or no charge. Video cameras or camcorders can be rented from local video stores, or purchased rather inexpensively. Some cell phones and computer notebooks can make videos and Flip Video cameras with costs starting online at $60.00 (www.amazon.com). Below are some tips for videotaping your valuables:

- ❑ Use techniques like panning, close-up shooting, and zooming for each possession.
- ❑ Make a video of all of your valuables by walking through your house room-by-room, including closets.
- ❑ For instructions from insurance industry experts on what you need to make note of in your home, check with your insurance agent.

General Preparation 97

- Pull valuables, such as furs and tapestries out of closets and onto beds for easier viewing.
- Lay jewelry and silver out on a table or countertop for close-up shots.
- Make sure all shots are in focus.
- Turn pottery and china over to film the artist's signature and trademarks.
- Narrate as you go, give purchase dates, place of purchase, and history of the items
- Go outside and record the exterior of the house and landscaping and hardscape as well.

Photographs and Digital Photographs

Another option for documenting valuables is to take color photographs of each item. Descriptions, dates, and prices can be written on the back of the photos. Update the photo inventory when adding to or subtracting from personal property. Be sure to have copies made, sent to your out-of-area contact, and stored in your emergency kit and safe deposit box with negatives or digital disc. Digital pictures can be loaded onto the computer and emailed, downloaded by printer or saved to a thumb or flash drive. Many home computers and tablets have Microsoft Windows Movie Maker already pre-loaded, and this is another way you can capture and import your photos into email, or burn home inventory onto CDs. Whatever form of documentation you use, always store a copy away from your home, so that regardless of the disaster, proof exists of your valuables.

Storage of Important Information

Now that the household inventory is complete and a videotape, negatives, or digital photographs have been created, a safe storage place should be established. If using a videotape, make several copies at the local photo shop. Store CDs, flash drives, videotapes, or digital disks in a safe deposit box or send to your out-of-area contact person. Make backup copies of everything and store them in your emergency kit, and send by mail or email to your out-of-area contact.

Include the following:
- ☐ Birth certificates
- ☐ Copies of driver's licenses
- ☐ Copies of social security cards
- ☐ Passport copies
- ☐ Death certificates
- ☐ Marriage certificate
- ☐ Divorce decree
- ☐ Child support orders
- ☐ Immunization records
- ☐ Vaccination records
- ☐ Signed medical releases
- ☐ "Do Not Resuscitate" orders
- ☐ Medical power of attorney
- ☐ Living wills
- ☐ Physicians' phone numbers
- ☐ Copies of important prescriptions
- ☐ Special allergy or blood medical needs information
- ☐ Deeds and contracts
- ☐ Car, boat, RV titles, license numbers, and VIN numbers
- ☐ Copies of mortgage statements
- ☐ Credit card companies and account numbers
- ☐ Bank, branch, checking/savings account numbers, contact, phone
- ☐ Certificates of deposit numbers, locations
- ☐ Safe Deposit information and key location
- ☐ Trust accounts, bank, branch, numbers, and phone
- ☐ Stocks and bonds

Neighborhood Plan

Utilize the national program Map Your Neighborhood (MYN) that can be found online for tips on how to organize an effort to prepare yourself and your neighbors for a disaster (www.earthquakeconference.org). Get to know your neighbors by setting up a meeting. Consider bringing in speakers from the Red Cross or local fire stations that will provide education on preparedness and emergency training. Ask the experts to show videos on disasters that may affect your area. Open a discussion on building emergency kits, and check with individuals and families to assure they have emergency supplies on hand or will take the next step to build a kit. Make an overall neighborhood plan including what special skills and equipment residents have. Pick a designated place for everyone to meet after a disaster and pinpoint where the local emergency staging area will be set up, in a school, recreation center, or church. Elect a block captain to be in charge and choose someone to serve as a back-up. Get proactive and check out how you can get certified as a first responder in your own neighborhood (www.citizencorps.gov) or through your local Neighborhood Emergency Team (NET).

Utilities and Hazards

Organize a system to help neighbors shut off their water, gas, and electricity. If a neighbor is disabled or incapacitated and can't shut off his gas, note that on your neighborhood list. Make sure everyone knows the location of their special shutoff tools and the correct shutoff procedures. As outlined in the household emergency plan, conduct a walk through, assess hazards, make punch lists, and help clean up and secure neighbor's homes. Review the instructions online (www.fema.gov/plan/prepare/utilityplan.shtm).

Signal Flag System

In your disaster plan, have a colored flag system to use on every front door in the neighborhood:

- Red means someone has been injured and needs help immediately.
- Yellow means some assistance is needed.
- White means everything is fine.

Tagging the doors with colored construction paper or ribbon broadcasts the status of every house. This system allows residents to quickly signal for help, and it assists neighbors and first responders to set rescue and medical priorities without physically going into each property. Enabling emergency responders to work more efficiently in a disaster promotes survival, and this is one good way to do so.

Resources and Experts

Make a neighborhood map that notes resident's skills, resources, expertise, and special needs. Note health professionals and other specialists like doctors, nurses, CPR, and first aid certified individuals, paramedics, firemen, police officers, plumbers, electricians, and contractors within your neighborhood. Note equipment resources such as ham radios, wireless email devices, portable generators, four-wheel drive vehicles, heavy equipment, and tools. In the event of a disaster, you'll know who to contact, allowing your neighborhood to work together as a true community.

The Elderly, Handicapped, and Infants

Prepare a list of the elderly, handicapped, pregnant women, and infants who will need help in a disaster. Check on emergency plans for your elderly neighbors. Find the United States toll-free number for each state for persons with speech

General Preparation 101

difficulty or who need speech-to speech translation (http://www.fcc.gov/cib/dro/sts.html). See online for additional information (www.fcc.gov/cgb/dro). For those who live in apartments, ask about the structural safety of the building. Ask about emergency plans and procedures, fire drills, sprinkler systems, monitored alarm systems, and fire equipment that could save lives in a disaster. Make the same inquiries at nursing homes and retirement centers in the area.

Helping Elderly and Handicapped Neighbors

Below are many ways that you can support your elderly or handicapped neighbors:

- ❑ Help elderly and handicapped neighbors store food, water, and supplies in their emergency kits.
- ❑ Test or install smoke alarms, and aid in assessing hazards.
- ❑ Make a punch list and form a neighborhood work crew as necessary.
- ❑ Cut down threatening tree limbs.
- ❑ Check fuse boxes and circuit breakers and bolt down hot water heaters.
- ❑ Bracket bookcases and heavy furniture to walls.
- ❑ If the neighbor's living situation is inadequate or unmanageable, talk to family members or social agencies that may be able to help.

The elderly or handicapped person may need care and supervision, and it is important to assess this before disaster strikes. In your own family, if your grandmother is isolated or ailing, consider bringing her into your home where she will be safe and looked after immediately following the disaster. That way, her daily needs can be met by household or family members until the emergency is over.

A more permanent option could also be finding a suitable care facility with trained medical personnel to look after elderly or handicapped loved ones. Check online (www.disabilitypreparedness.gov) for safe and secure tips to help people with disabilities.

Pet Plan

There are a number of steps to take for the well-being and survival of pets, livestock, or farm animals. First, make sure your animals have some type of identification so they can be returned should they get lost during a disaster. Herds of cattle should be branded, and cats and dogs should wear collars with I.D. tags attached. Include the pet's name and your name, address, email, and telephone or cell number on the tag. For the animal's protection, pet vaccinations should be kept current. House pets and rare or valuable animals can be implanted with computer chip tracking devices to make the search easier. This can be done by a veterinarian. Check the resources at the Center for Disease Control and Prevention and online (www.bt.cdc.gov/disasters/petprotect.asp and www.ready.gov/america/getakit/pets.html).

In a disaster, familiar scents and landmarks may change and cause disorientation for animals. If pet(s) become lost, it will help to have a current snapshot to show others and post on bulletin boards at grocery stores and veterinarians' offices. Another way to help locate pets after a disaster is to be aware of the places they like to hide around the house or in the yard. This is particularly true of cats. Go online for more details on ASPCA tips for pet care (http://www.aspca.org/pet-care/disaster-preparedness).

Below are more tips for pet safety in the event of a disaster:
- ❑ Keep leashes and pet carriers big enough to hold the

General Preparation 103

animals on hand so animals can be contained and calmed at home.
❑ Put a bowl for water, a towel, and a litter box in the carrier.
❑ Throw an extra towel or blanket over the carrier once your pet is settled in to calm the animal.
❑ Store pet photos, supplies, food, water, spare leashes, and collars with your emergency kit.
❑ Pet's health and vaccination records, medications, special diet needs, and feeding schedules should go in the kit too.
❑ In a disaster, pets and other animals are likely to become frightened and agitated. Approach animals cautiously as they may be aggressive.
❑ Animals returning home after a disaster should be contained or leashed before getting close to people.
❑ Be prepared for pet readjustment periods of up to several days.

Be aware Red Cross emergency shelters will not allow animals, due to health and safety laws. Make alternate plans and arrange staying with your pet at friends or relatives outside of the immediate disaster area. Pet-friendly motels and hotels will allow pets for a small fee. Call ahead for restrictions on breeds, sizes, and number of animals. Reservations for both lodging and boarding facilities may also be needed. Your local veterinarian might recommend a good kennel as well. Some holding areas for pets, livestock, and farm animals will be set up after the disaster via emergency services. This information will be broadcast on the radio following an event. Read about animal microchip implanting and how animal recovery works with these chips (http://www.humanesociety.org/animals/resources/tips/microchips.html).

School Plan

When natural or man-made disasters strike, schools are often affected. Because blizzards, earthquakes, fires, or nuclear plant reactor accidents can happen at any time, knowing the school plan is an important part of disaster preparedness. In recent years, violent shootings by students on school campuses have made international headlines, raised safety concerns, and brought to light additional reasons to have a disaster plan in place. Checking on the emergency preparedness and evacuation plans for your children's school is a basic step. Current laws require school site councils to have a safety plan in place. Present this list of questions to your school's PTA, administrator, or site council:

- Has the building recently passed an official structural, fire, and safety inspection?
- Is the building earthquake safe? If it is an older building, have seismic retrofitting adaptations been made?
- Does the school district have a policy on disasters?
- Is there a multi-hazard emergency plan in place? Does the plan cover a minimum of 48 hours after a strike?
- Is the plan reviewed every year for any needed changes? Who reviews the plan and what are their qualifications or certifications?
- Can parents take part in emergency planning and organization?
- Will notices of emergency and disaster preparation exercises be sent to parents?
- Will the school send parents complete descriptions of the exercises so they can practice drills with children at home?
- Are certificates of completion of the emergency and disaster training given out to students?

General Preparation

- ❏ What are the limits of the liability, medical, and insurance coverage of the schools?
- ❏ Is the school away from the flood plain? If a flood occurs, is the school covered by flood insurance?
- ❏ Does the school have an up-to-date sprinkler and fire alarm system? Is the system monitored?
- ❏ Are fire escapes in good working order?
- ❏ Are regular fire drills conducted for students and teachers?
- ❏ Does the building have basement shelter stocked with emergency food, water, supplies, first aid kit, and an EBS radio?
- ❏ Is an inventory and rotation record kept of supplies?
- ❏ Is there a backup generator to run the school's heating and electricity if power goes out?
- ❏ Is there a "shelter in place" plan with students kept inside the school until picked up by a household or family member?
- ❏ If a parent is unable to pick a child up, can another adult be authorized by the parent with a phone call, fax, or email to the school?
- ❏ Following an emergency, will school authorities send children home on their own?
- ❏ If phone lines are down in a crisis, what is the backup communication system? Are two-way radios or wireless email available?
- ❏ How does the school communicate with students, first responder agencies, and the news media in a disaster?
- ❏ How and when will parents be contacted during or after a disaster?
- ❏ How will parents be kept up-to-date on emergency developments? Is there a hotline to call, text messaging, email, or Twitter set up?

- Does the school require parent's emergency phone numbers to be updated in writing? Can a phone call, text, fax, or email be used?
- What are the evacuation plans and procedures?
- Where are the emergency exits located? Is there a map of exits and escape routes displayed in a main hallway?
- Is a map of the evacuation routes available for parents to study?
- Are students walked or bused through the actual evacuation routes during regular drills? How often are disaster drills conducted?
- Have several alternate evacuation routes been created in case any roads are blocked?
- How will bus drivers be contacted if evacuation is necessary? Do they carry two-way radios, cell phones, or pagers?
- How and when will parents be notified of evacuation?
- Do bus drivers practice driving the evacuation routes?
- Are emergency supplies, equipment, and first aid kits kept on school buses in case sheltering on the bus is necessary?
- Do the buses carry traction devices on board in case of snowy or icy weather?
- Is locker or other storage space available at the school for student's personal emergency kit?
- What will happen if shots are fired in the school? Is a lockdown plan in place?
- What will happen in the case of a bomb threat or explosion? Will parents be notified at the time of the threat?
- How will law enforcement officials be contacted in case of a shooting, and who will assume command?
- Are drills practiced for a weaponized attack?

General Preparation

- ☐ Is someone in charge trained in the Incident Command System?
- ☐ If a crisis happens before school, will students be contacted and told not to come to school?
- ☐ Can bus drivers be warned on their two-way radio, cell phones, or pagers?
- ☐ If nuclear substances, chemical, or biological agents are deployed by terrorists, how will they be detected?
- ☐ What medical personnel will be standing by? Does the school nurse have adequate supplies to treat a lot of injuries at once?
- ☐ Are nurses and teachers trained to identify, treat, and report incidents involving biological and chemical agents? What are the procedures?
- ☐ If a large number of students experience vomiting and high fever during a possible chemical release are anecdotes readily available?
- ☐ Would a high incidence of flu during the off-season raise a red flag for staff personnel? What procedures would they follow?
- ☐ How will viral or bacterial outbreaks be contained to keep them from becoming epidemics?
- ☐ In case of sudden, high numbers of illness or deaths, what will the school do to treat the outbreak?
- ☐ Will vaccines and antibiotics be available quickly? Where are they kept and how are they transported?
- ☐ Do nursing staff have immediate access to student's medical records and who is at high risk for toxic reactions to vaccines?
- ☐ In the case of a biological attack, how would isolation and quarantine be handled?
- ☐ Besides anthrax and smallpox, what other viruses or bacterial agents are anticipated?

- How and when would parents be notified of such an incident?
- In the event of nuclear or chemical attack, is there a decontamination plan in place? Could locker room showers be used?
- What nearby medical facility, military base, or hospital could be used for decontamination or quarantine?
- Has school staff contacted nearby chemical, hazardous waste, and nuclear power plants for information and training?
- Has this information been integrated into the school plan?
- Do bus drivers practice the hazardous facilities' evacuation routes during regular drills?
- Are regular FEMA drills conducted on the regulated emergency plans for nuclear and chemical facilities?
- Are both sheltering in place and evacuation covered in these plans?
- What other nearby facility besides the school could be used for shelter in case the school is too badly damaged to be safe?

Workplace Plan

The average worker spends at least eight hours a day, or a third of all waking time on the job. Some people even work two jobs. Does your employer have an emergency plan? Do you know what to do after a disaster strikes your place of work? If a disaster strikes while you are at work, are you prepared to be confined to the office for up to 72 hours afterwards? Does your office emergency kit have what you need to "shelter in place" at work for three days or more?

Get more information online about sheltering in place (www.osha.gov/SLTC/etools/evacuation/shelterinplace.

General Preparation

html). Plans will vary based on where you work. You can also view our website for tips on putting together a business continuity plan to get your company back to work after a disaster (www.naturaldisastersbook.com). Amanda Ripley's harrowing account of those who survived in the World Trade Center's twin towers on 9/11 reveals that most survivors went on autopilot and put their escape plan into action (www.amandaripley.com). Ask the following questions of your workplace security department to ensure that your office or jobsite is prepared in the event of a disaster:

- ❑ Does your company have an emergency plan?
- ❑ Does your company have a business continuity plan for recovering after a disaster?
- ❑ Can your company send out an emergency notification to you in a disaster?
- ❑ Is there a way for you to send in a notification to your company that you are "ok" in a disaster?
- ❑ Has the building you work in recently passed a structural safety, fire, and earthquake inspection?
- ❑ Is the structure earthquake safe? If the building is older, has it been retrofitted to meet seismic codes?
- ❑ Has the site been inspected for hazards? Have required corrections been made?
- ❑ Have precautions been taken to avoid injuries such as securing heavy objects to the structure?
- ❑ Is the company complying with OSHA workplace safety regulations?
- ❑ Are regular disaster preparedness and fire drills conducted for all employees and management?
- ❑ Is the sprinkler system in working order? Have fire escapes been inspected?
- ❑ What responsibilities will workers and managers have if a disaster strikes when they are on the job?

- What are your disaster related duties? Will you be on call if a disaster strikes while you are at home?
- Have leaders been chosen to be in charge of each floor of the building? What are the duties of department heads?
- Have those in charge had emergency preparedness training and been certified in first aid and CPR?
- What backup and security measures have been taken to protect computer databases, files, documents, and information systems?
- Is an evacuation plan in place, and are alternate routes mapped out? Is the map displayed or available by computer or mobile device where everyone can see it?
- Are emergency supplies, food, and water stored in a shelter on-site? Is an EBS radio available?
- Is storage available on-site for workers' personal disaster kits?
- Does your office or workplace have a list of employees with special needs who will need assistance in an emergency?
- Are there special alerts for hearing or visually impaired employees, vendors, and customers?
- Are some emergency exits equipped with wheelchair ramps or lifts? What help will be provided for mobility-impaired individuals?
- How will disabled employees be helped in case of a disaster?

Disaster preparedness for businesses should include a business continuity plan to survive a disaster. Emergency notification systems exist that can push out a message to all employees on their computers and mobile devices in the event of a crisis. The incident could be anything from extreme weather to a terrorist attack, but you could be notified and you could respond "I'm ok" using technological systems available today. Ask your employer about their disaster recovery plans. View online how emergency notification systems can be sent in multiple formats in a disaster to as few as two to more than 20,000 employees until they are reached and can respond (http://www.sendwordnow.com).

Church Plan

Many different religions exist in the world and churches, parishes, temples, synagogues, and mosques often represent stability and a safe haven in a crisis. When calamity strikes, many will seek help at these neighborhood and community centers. Consult with your local religious leaders to get the necessary information in case of a disaster. You can review the religious agencies worldwide that help in disasters (http://www.disastercenter.com/agency.htm). These agencies are often the first to arrive in a disaster, and their efforts many times exceed the stymied attempts by government agencies, as evidenced in Hurricane Katrina. Below is a list of questions to present to the priest, rabbi, or cleric at your particular place of worship:

- ❑ Has the church passed a building, safety, and fire inspection? Have the cited conditions been upgraded to meet code?
- ❑ If the building is older, has it been retrofitted for protection against earthquakes?
- ❑ Has an inspection been conducted to identify exterior hazards, such as trees that could fall on the building?
- ❑ Is it possible to use the church as a shelter?
- ❑ Could the building be used as a quarantine facility?
- ❑ Are emergency training, first aid, and CPR classes offered to the community in the church facility?
- ❑ Could neighborhood planning and organizational meetings be held in a Sunday school classroom or in the worship space?

- ❏ Has an Emergency and Disaster Preparedness Committee been appointed?
- ❏ What interaction with other churches does the preparedness committee have? Is the support network being utilized effectively?
- ❏ Have members of the clergy taken emergency preparedness and first aid training? Do they know CPR?
- ❏ Do church leaders know where fire exits, ladders, and hoses are? Do they know how to use firefighting tools?
- ❏ Are regular fire drills and disaster drills conducted with the congregation?
- ❏ Does the church have a working sprinkler system?
- ❏ Do leaders and staff know where utility shutoff valves and tools are located?
- ❏ Do a number of people know where the electric fuse box or circuit breaker is, and how and when to restore or shut off the electricity?
- ❏ Are fresh fuses available in case of a power outage? Has the circuit breaker box passed an inspection or been upgraded to meet code?
- ❏ Have exits and evacuation routes been planned and practiced? Are alternate routes mapped out in case some roads are blocked?
- ❏ Is there a list of congregation members according to special needs and their ability to help out?
- ❏ Is it known who has a power generator, who is a doctor, and who is in a wheel chair?
- ❏ Is a stockpile of emergency supplies, food, and water stored in a secure place on-site? Does it include an EBS radio?
- ❏ How will emergency information, disaster warnings, or evacuation announcements be relayed to church members in a disaster?

General Preparation 113

- ❏ How will household and family members be contacted if their relatives, children, or spouses are injured or killed in a disaster?
- ❏ Is there a basement to take shelter in if a tornado, hurricane, or other calamity strikes during a service?
- ❏ Will the church leaders be available after a disaster to offer crisis counseling?
- ❏ What other assistance will be offered? Will hot meals be available? Are shelter and first aid available at the church?

Bank Plan

An access to funds and to safety deposit boxes for important papers including wills, appraisals, insurance policies, trust deeds, mortgages, and financial and investment information will be very important after a disaster. Some suggested questions to ask your bank manager are as follows:

- ❏ Has the bank passed a recent building, fire, and safety inspection?
- ❏ Does the building meet seismic codes in case of an earthquake?
- ❏ If the building is older, have seismic retrofitting adaptations been made?
- ❏ Is the building away from the flood plain? If a flood occurs, will insurance cover it?
- ❏ What are the bank's emergency plans and evacuation procedures?
- ❏ Are emergency, fire, and disaster drills conducted for all employees, management, and security personnel on a regular basis?
- ❏ Who is capable of assuming command in case of an armed robbery, an explosion, or a bomb threat?
- ❏ Are lockdown procedures in place? How will authorities and police be notified?

- ❑ How will the money be safeguarded? What are the security procedures, checks and balances?
- ❑ Is the bank federally insured? What are the dollar limits for each account and safety deposit box?
- ❑ How will the bank operate after a disaster? How can accounts be accessed after a disaster?
- ❑ How and when will account holders be contacted regarding their accounts and investments after a disaster?

Retirement Facility Plan

Just as it is important to know the school and work place emergency preparedness plans for your loved ones, it is also critical to find out about the plans in place where your parents, grandparents, elderly friends, and retired neighbors live. Scores of retirement facilities are now available to meet the housing and healthcare needs of a rapidly growing elderly population. There are all types of living arrangements available for older people. The variety spans active retirement communities with complete recreational facilities, condominium developments of all sizes, cooperative associations, group homes for the disabled, assisted living residences with hospital wings, and traditional nursing homes with around the clock care.

Some housing communities and condominium associations are designated specifically to serve tenants and owners over the age of 55, while others start admitting people at age 65. Read a report on the findings of Nursing Home Evacuation Plans across the country (http://www.ncbi.nlm.nih.gov/PMC/articles). Learn about evacuation and relocation plans for any emergency, from a fire or flood to an earthquake or toxic chemical release. Housing in a retirement or nursing home is regulated by state and Federal agencies. Meeting building codes, passing regular inspections,

General Preparation

and having emergency and evacuation plans are components of compliance. Plans must be tested. If the facility has been cited in violation of the requirements, a resident may want to consider moving. Check the National Center on Elder Abuse for resources and tips (www.ncea.aoa.gov).

Any unsafe living situation will need to be changed. Your mother-in-law's apartment may work fine with only a few minor additions like grab bars in the shower and 10-year smoke alarms in the bedrooms, but if she lives in an older building that does not meet current fire and seismic codes, relocating her may be necessary. Moving to a newer, more up-to-date apartment closer to family may be the best solution. Following are some suggested questions to ask retirement facility managers:

- ❏ Has the facility recently passed a building, safety, and fire inspection?
- ❏ Has the building met earthquake codes? If it is an older facility, have seismic retrofitting adaptations been made?
- ❏ Is a Red Cross or Fire Department expert scheduled to give a class on emergency preparedness, first aid, and CPR training for residents, patients, and relatives?
- ❏ Is the staff trained and certified in first aid and CPR?
- ❏ Have doctors and nurses been trained and certified as emergency responders?
- ❏ Has the staff had disaster preparedness and drills?
- ❏ What qualifications, training, and certification do the people in charge have?
- ❏ Are disaster and fire drills conducted for staff and residents?
- ❏ Are sprinkler systems and fire escapes well maintained?
- ❏ How and when will relatives be contacted after the disaster?
- ❏ How comprehensive is the facility's insurance and

- liability coverage, and how high are the limits for medical coverage?
- Is the building away from the flood plain? If not, is a flood insurance policy in place?
- Does the building have a well-stocked basement shelter with emergency supplies, food, water, and EBS radios?
- Are two-way radios and wireless email devices available in case phone lines are down?
- Are back-up medical supplies and equipment stored on-site?
- Is a back-up generator available to run heat, air conditioning, lights, and medical equipment in case of a power outage?
- What are the evacuation plans and routes?
- How and when will spouses and relatives be contacted in case of evacuation?
- Where are the emergency exits located, and what are the escape and evacuation routes?
- What transportation will be used to evacuate?
- Is medical staff trained in identifying symptoms of illness from viral, bacterial, and chemical agents?
- If necessary, how soon can anecdotes and vaccines be delivered and administered?
- What containment and quarantine procedures are in place?
- Are medical personnel qualified to diagnose and treat radiation sickness?
- If this is a nursing home or an assisted living facility with a hospital wing on-site, how will patients be evacuated?
- What facility will evacuees be relocated to? How do the medical resources of the new facility compare to the present one?

General Preparation

- ❏ What precautions and procedures are in place to safeguard the blood supply?
- ❏ Do patients store their own blood before surgery? If a patient is chemically sensitive, can the blood be contained in glass bottles?
- ❏ How are controlled substances stored and handled?
- ❏ If a resident needs off-site hospitalization, what transportation will be used?
- ❏ Does the facility have its own ambulance, bus, or van?
- ❏ Are ambulances and life flight helicopters readily available in medical emergencies?
- ❏ Do residents of rural areas need special medical transportation insurance?
- ❏ Is a policy or membership to an ambulance or life flight service available in rural areas? What is the cost?
- ❏ If the patient is a veteran required to receive VA paid medical benefits at a veteran's hospital, does insurance cover an ambulance?
- ❏ Is life flight insurance available for VA patients? What is the cost?
- ❏ In a disaster, will the VA patient be able to receive paid medical help at a reachable civilian hospital?
- ❏ What notification will be given to emergency contacts and family when a resident is hospitalized on or off-site?
- ❏ Are signed consent forms for medical treatment needed in advance? Can the forms be faxed or emailed?
- ❏ Does the facility use the Red Cross Vial of Life forms to keep tabs on patient's vital medical information?
- ❏ Is legal advice available on Medical Power of Attorney, Advance Directives, and Health Care Representatives?
- ❏ Are the legal and medical forms available on-site at the facility, at the hospital, or online?
- ❏ Are "Do Not Resuscitate" orders kept on file?

❑ Are "Physician's Orders for Life Sustaining Treatment" kept on file?
❑ How often does the staff reevaluate residents' medical and legal information, and reassess their needs and type of care?

Supplies Storage

Designate household members to be responsible for gathering food, and storing water and other supplies. Check the kitchen pantry for foods that will keep well in storage, such as canned goods and freeze-dried camping meals. Include foods that you like to eat, and stock comfort foods like tins of saltine crackers, packets of trail mix, dried beef jerky, peanut butter bars, bricks of ramen noodles, and jars of pasta sauce. You can throw in cans of soft cheese, tuna, spam, olives, pork and beans, peaches, pineapple, and applesauce for good measure. This will make survival much more bearable and give you tasty treats to look forward to. Plan for a three-day supply of food and water at a minimum, and extend that to a three-week supply if room permits. Also remember to store food, water, and supplies for pets.

Food Storage

In a disaster, if you can stay home, eat perishable food from the refrigerator first. Consume the freshest foods and then frozen foods over a period of four to seven days. For stored items, rotate and replace stored foods noting expiration dates. When purchasing food, be aware that some discount food stores sell items that are close to their expiration dates, if not already expired. Also read labels to check sodium content as salty foods can make you thirsty and you will want to conserve your limited supply of water.

Water Storage

Store water in unbreakable plastic jugs and write the date of storage on the bottle. Replace the water every six months to keep the supply fresh. Remember to allow for one gallon of water per person, per day. Half a gallon is for drinking and the other half is for washing. More water may be needed if you live in a hot, dry climate.

When storing water in recycled containers, clean quart or liter containers thoroughly. Heavy jugs are preferred since the lighter bottles tend to break and crack. Adding sodium hypochlorite can extend the shelf life of water up to five years. Another method to extend the water's shelf life is to block any light by covering bottles with black, plastic trash bags. If storing the bottles in an unheated garage or a car trunk, do not fill fully. Leave a little space at the top for the water to expand during cold winter conditions or freezing. This will eliminate the problem of spillage, water loss, and mildew infestation on clothing or camping supplies stored nearby.

If using polyethylene plastic containers, be aware that they can absorb toxic vapors especially from hydrocarbons. To be safe, store the bottles of water well away from pesticides, gasoline, or kerosene. Vinyl containers can also leak toxins. Do not drink water from waterbeds, garbage cans or bleach bottles. Do not refill empty milk or detergent bottles, as toxic effects may result.

Buying commercially bottled water requires less effort and time, and it ensures longer shelf life. Heavy-duty five gallon bottles can last anywhere from five to 10 years. Do not store plastic water jugs on concrete floors as they can absorb chemical toxins. Smaller commercial bottles of water expire more quickly. Other supplies to gather are personal health and hygiene articles, camping equipment, tools, pet supplies, and first aid items. Camping equipment may be the best immediate source of shelter after the disaster. Being able to camp may allow you to stay on your own property and monitor the situation. Be sure to include any special prescription medications in your first aid kit and update these medications at least once a year. As a general rule, when old supplies are discarded, they should be replaced.

Decide where you're going to store emergency supplies and put everything in one safe, accessible place. A cool, dark area in a garage, a closet, basement, or under a bed are all good storage locations. This is also the time to collect supplies for small emergency kits going to the office and school or daycare. Distribute the kits accordingly. Emergency kits should also be placed in car trunks. For evacuation purposes, supply containers should be easy to move. Backpacks, coolers on wheels, and garbage cans on wheels all work efficiently and provide easy transport.

Lists of Supplies to Store

Hygiene and Sanitation List

Add the following to your emergency supply list to meet hygiene and sanitation needs for daily, personal use:

- Toothbrush, toothpaste, floss
- Spare dentures, partial plates, retainers
- Shampoo, lotion, sunblock
- Comb, brush, mirror
- Bar soap, washcloths
- Shaving kit, deodorant
- Toilet paper in plastic container
- Five gallon bucket with lid and bag of sand for makeshift toilet

General Preparation

- ❑ Plastic dishpan
- ❑ Bath towels
- ❑ Sanitary pads, tampons
- ❑ Lime powder for latrine disinfectant
- ❑ Eyedropper, eyewash
- ❑ Large plastic garbage bags and ties
- ❑ Plastic bucket with tight lid for toilet
- ❑ Garbage bags and ties for waste disposal
- ❑ Portable camp toilet
- ❑ Liquid bleach, sodium hypochlorite
- ❑ One gallon of washing water per day, per person

Baby Supply/Hygiene and Sanitation List

- ❑ Formula, pure water
- ❑ Bottles, disposable liners, and nipples
- ❑ Powdered milk
- ❑ Pacifier
- ❑ Baby cream, lotion, powder
- ❑ Medications
- ❑ Towel, washcloth
- ❑ Baby wipes
- ❑ Disposable diapers
- ❑ Plastic bags and ties for waste disposal
- ❑ Small garbage can with tight lid
- ❑ Warm blanket, pillow
- ❑ Warm clothing

Camping Equipment List

In a disaster, temporary shelter facilities may not be reachable or available. Hotels and motels may be full or unable to take your pets. In any event, a suggested list of camping supplies should be stored for your comfort, whether camping at home or elsewhere. Work from the following suggested list by checking your home items first to see what you have on hand. What you don't have on hand can be purchased at most big box stores or camping outlets.

- ❑ Foil space blankets
- ❑ Wool blankets
- ❑ Change of clothes for everyone
- ❑ Sweat clothes, long underwear, socks
- ❑ Rain gear, warm jackets
- ❑ Sturdy shoes or hiking boots
- ❑ Shorts and t-shirts
- ❑ Sunglasses and sunblock
- ❑ Hats and gloves
- ❑ Sleeping bags and foam mats
- ❑ Tent, stakes, tarp, and cover
- ❑ Three or more tarps to cover supplies
- ❑ Matches in a waterproof container
- ❑ Multifunctional camping knife
- ❑ Whistle
- ❑ Mess kits, plastic or paper plates, cups, and bowls
- ❑ Plastic utensils
- ❑ Manual can opener, Swiss army knife
- ❑ Ice chest
- ❑ Propane stove, propane fuel
- ❑ Sterno stove
- ❑ Hibachi grill, charcoal
- ❑ Axe, shovel, pickaxe
- ❑ Fluorescent or battery-powered lantern
- ❑ Extra alkaline batteries
- ❑ Flashlight and separate alkaline batteries
- ❑ Hand crank flashlight and hand crank cell phone charger
- ❑ Portable radio or TV
- ❑ Emergency broadcast radio

General Preparation 123

- Bungee cords, 50–75 feet of Nylon cord, rope
- Local map
- Postcards, pens, stamps, books, and periodicals
- Bucket
- ABC fire extinguisher
- Pepper spray or mace
- Windup clock
- Toys, games, puzzles, paperbacks, notebooks, pens

Store these items together in a large rolling garbage can where you can get to it in an emergency.

Tools and Materials List

You will need tools and materials to dislodge rubble, shore up windows, and make necessary repairs. Work from the following suggested list:

- Second-story high ladder
- Wheelbarrow
- Rake
- Long-handle, round-point shovel
- Chainsaw
- Pruning saw
- Claw hammer
- Sledge hammer
- Nails and screws
- Set of crescent wrenches or adjustable wrench
- Pliers
- Phillips screwdriver
- Flat-end screwdriver
- Heavy duty staple gun and staples
- Electrician's tape, duct tape
- Plastic sheeting to cover broken windows
- Sandbags, bucket
- Plywood and boards

- Water-main wrench
- Gas-main wrench (or four-in-one tool)
- Crowbar and bolt cutters

Store these items in your garage or an outside shed for easy access.

Food List

Storage of sufficient food and water is essential for survival. Without water, dehydration and death can occur. Thirst is the primary need, and food is secondary. Shop carefully and choose foods such as canned goods that will not spoil or need refrigeration. Look for foods with at least a six-month expiration date and store them in a dark, dry area with a temperature less than 70 degrees Fahrenheit. Avoid salty foods that will increase thirst.

It is very important psychologically to have something good tasting to eat in the midst of disaster's chaos and transition. Plan menus ahead and eliminate leftovers with one meal serving sizes. Food products that come in large quantities can be split up into numerous small plastic bags. Reduce exposure to oxygen and moisture, and protect from pest and rodent contamination by keeping food in sealed containers. Paper packages may be placed in metal cans and sealed shut. Freeze-dried foods can be found online (www.nitro-pak.com).

Food and water should be rotated and replaced annually. It is recommended that you try these foods *before* packing them away for later use. Rotate out your stock and make a meal under the best-case scenario to see if you actually like this type of food and would eat if comfortably. The following food preparation list will help you know what to store in the event of a disaster:

- Water: one gallon per person, per day
- Freeze-dried meals

General Preparation 125

- ❏ Dried fruit, raisins
- ❏ Nuts, granola, or power bars
- ❏ Canned fish
- ❏ Canned soup, chili, and beans in ready-to-eat containers
- ❏ Canned vegetables and fruits
- ❏ Crackers, cookies
- ❏ Cereal, oatmeal
- ❏ Peanut butter, honey, jam
- ❏ Powdered or canned milk
- ❏ Baby food in jars, canned juice, powdered milk, or formula
- ❏ Cans of vegetable or fruit juice
- ❏ Instant drink mixes to add to water
- ❏ Pet food and water

Suggested Menus

There are a number of cookbooks on the market for menu planning without power. A funny one is *Apocalypse Chow, How to Eat Well When the Power Goes Out* by Jon Robertson and Robin Robertson (www.amazon.com). It's full of recipes like Last Resort Lasagna and Puttanesca in a Pinch, as well as Use-it-Up Minestrone Soup.

First Aid List

First aid kits may be purchased from the Red Cross, big box stores, AAA, online, at a local pharmacy, or at a camping supply store. You can gather many items from your existing medicine chest or from camping supplies. *Helpful tip:* storing prescription medications in the refrigerator will keep medicine fresher, longer. If shopping for first aid supplies, check expiration dates. Learning first aid will promote self-reliance and increase survival odds. Check supplies every six months to make sure items are not leaking or wet, and replace as necessary to keep them freshly stocked. Take a smaller version of the kit on trips and outings. Work from the following suggested list:

- ☐ Red Cross first aid manual
- ☐ Water purification tablets
- ☐ Sterile surgical gloves
- ☐ Aspirin or non-aspirin pain reliever
- ☐ Rubbing alcohol
- ☐ Bar soap
- ☐ Hydrogen peroxide
- ☐ Cortisone cream
- ☐ Vaseline
- ☐ Wash and wipes
- ☐ Insect repellent
- ☐ Calamine lotion
- ☐ Boric acid
- ☐ Cough syrup
- ☐ Benadryl
- ☐ Laxatives
- ☐ Sterile cotton balls, Q-Tips, eyedropper
- ☐ Instant ice packs
- ☐ Container of assorted band-aids
- ☐ 2x4 rolls of sterile gauze bandages, tape
- ☐ Triangle, ace, and butterfly bandages
- ☐ 4x4 gauze pads
- ☐ Ace bandages
- ☐ Splints
- ☐ Strips of sheets or pillow cases
- ☐ Scissors, tweezers
- ☐ Tissues
- ☐ Thread, needle, safety pins
- ☐ Vitamins, homeopathic remedies
- ☐ Current prescription medications
- ☐ Heart medications

General Preparation 127

- ☐ Insulin
- ☐ High blood pressure medicine
- ☐ Safety goggles, backup prescription eyeglasses
- ☐ Pocket mask with disposable mouth valve
- ☐ Signed medical release forms, physicians' directives
- ☐ Medical power of attorney forms
- ☐ DNR forms

Pet Supply List

Below is a list of items to store for your pets. Your veterinarian may have additional recommendations. Red Cross Shelters do not accept pets due to health and safety regulations. Service animals such as seeing-eye dogs are exceptions. Be sure to work from the following suggested list:

- ☐ Minimum three gallons of water per pet
- ☐ Pet carriers, leashes, collars, and extras
- ☐ Litter box
- ☐ Sand or pet litter, litter bags
- ☐ Canned or dried pet food in closed container (preferably their regular food)
- ☐ Feeding schedule
- ☐ Health and vaccination records required for admittance to emergency pet areas
- ☐ List of boarding kennels and phone numbers
- ☐ Veterinarian phone number
- ☐ Emergency shelters that take pets, phone numbers
- ☐ Motels and hotels accepting pets, phone numbers
- ☐ Special needs information with instructions
- ☐ Pet prescription medications
- ☐ Manual can opener
- ☐ Bowls, water pails
- ☐ Towel, blanket, brush
- ☐ Disinfectants, flea powder
- ☐ Hydrogen peroxide to use for wounds or poisonings

Personal Items List

You will want to have important information on hand in order to expedite your personal affairs. Insurance policy, medical data, financial information, and your out-of-area contact information should all be on hand. Carry emergency phone numbers as well. Use the following list to draw from, and put this into your emergency kit in case you need to evacuate:

- Cash in small bills, average of $500 per household
- Insurance policy
- Appraisal
- Documentation of home improvements
- Fireproof strong box
- Car titles
- Vehicle license numbers (VIN)
- Loan documents
- Mortgage paperwork
- Credit card account numbers, phone numbers
- Family photos
- Contact person information
- Emergency information
- Identification, birth certificates
- Household and family medical information
- Tax returns
- Videotape, CD, digital disc, flash drive of personal possessions
- Car key, house key, safe deposit key

Car Emergency Kit List

When traveling to and from work or on short trips or vacations, you will need to be prepared. Disasters happen anytime and anywhere. Always carry rain gear and warm, protective clothing and shoes. Be ready to meet the

General Preparation

challenges of changing weather conditions and other sudden emergencies. Evacuation may be required, so keep at least half a tank of gas in the car just in case. Another possibility is being stranded and having to shelter in the car. Even if you are renting a car, you should have a small emergency kit with you and always carry water. In order to be self-sufficient until rescue crews arrive, keep the following suggested items in the trunk of your car and glove box:

- ❑ First aid kit
- ❑ Two or three gallons of water (leave two inches at top in case of freezing)
- ❑ Flares
- ❑ Flashlight, separate alkaline batteries
- ❑ Cellular phone and crank charger
- ❑ Portable radio or EBS radio
- ❑ Separate alkaline batteries
- ❑ Compass, road map marked with shelter locations
- ❑ Extra prescription eyeglasses, sunglasses
- ❑ Necessary prescription medications
- ❑ Identification, medical alert tags
- ❑ Matches in dry, airtight container
- ❑ Camping shovel
- ❑ ABC fire extinguisher
- ❑ Heavy work gloves
- ❑ Heavy shoes
- ❑ Warm clothing
- ❑ Shorts and t-shirts
- ❑ Rain gear, umbrella
- ❑ Tarp, blankets (wool, solar), bright signal cloth
- ❑ Bungee cords
- ❑ Canned food, nuts, juices
- ❑ Power bars, beef jerky
- ❑ Crackers, peanut butter

- ❏ Manual can opener, utensils, cup
- ❏ Tire chains, towing rope
- ❏ Battery cables
- ❏ Help sign or paper and pencil to write a message on
- ❏ Window scraper
- ❏ Emergency contact person information and plan
- ❏ Cash and phone card
- ❏ Large bucket for emergency toilet, toilet paper
- ❏ Paperback book or puzzle

Office Emergency Kit List

In the event of a disaster while at work, plan on being stranded at the office for up to three days as a worst-case scenario and be sure to have sufficient supplies for that time frame. Services may be cut off in the event of a disaster and roads may not be accessible, so it's best to assume you will spend up to three days away from home. Walking may be necessary to return home. You may need the following:

- ❏ Three gallons of bottled water
- ❏ Cash and phone card
- ❏ Identification
- ❏ Personal hygiene items—toothbrush, hairbrush, shampoo
- ❏ Emergency contact person information and plan
- ❏ Flashlight, separate alkaline batteries
- ❏ Portable radio, separate alkaline batteries
- ❏ Canned food, nuts, juice, manual can opener, utensils, cup
- ❏ Rain gear
- ❏ Warm clothing, heavy gloves, and shoes
- ❏ First aid kit
- ❏ Prescription medications
- ❏ Sleeping bag, mat, blanket

Natural Disasters

All regions of the world are subordinate to nature's powerful forces. Natural disasters are as much a part of life now as they have been in the past and will be in the future. Historically, these natural phenomena have peaked in recurring monumental events that have changed and molded the earth over eons of time. Earthquakes and volcanic eruptions raised islands, sculpted mountains, and molded coastlines and lava plains. Floods covered the landscape and altered its shape and vegetation. Hurricanes washed away shorelines, driving torrents of rain and ocean waters inland. Wildfires swept through forests and burned them down, thinning trees and enriching soil.

From the beginning of civilization, the destructive powers of nature have inspired awe and fear. Humans living on the land have reckoned with the challenge of nature, often resulting in the survival of only the fittest. At their worst, natural disasters wreak havoc. They inflict catastrophic destruction on communities and their citizens; bringing death, injury, and property damage totaling billions of dollars.

EARTHQUAKES

Earthquakes have struck without warning at every hour and in every season all over the world. Devastating quakes have rocked China, France, Portugal, Japan, Peru, Sumatra, Chile, Haiti, and the United States in Alaska, Hawaii, Oregon, and California. Earthquakes are raging catastrophic events which can cause enormous damage in a minute or less. On March 11, 2011 the worldwide news media captivated a global audience with extensive coverage of a magnitude 9.0 quake that embattled Japan, spun off a tsunami that hit 50 countries and caused a nuclear plant meltdown the size of Chernobyl. On the same day, a 5.8 magnitude quake struck China. Decades earlier, the San Francisco Loma Prieta or "World Series" quake of 1989 measured a magnitude of 7.1 and lasted just ten seconds. It cost $10 billion in damages.

Enormous loss of life can result from one of these deadly and powerful seismic disasters. A magnitude 10.0 quake devastated Sumatra in 2004 and left 160,000 dead. In 2010, a 7.0 quake lambasted Haiti. The toll was over 200,000 dead. Just a month later, an 8.8 quake rocked Chili. The turbo force sped up the Earth's rotation, altered its axis, and shortened our days. The United States Geological Service tracks the magnitude of earthquakes worldwide on a daily basis, which you can see on its website (www.earthquake.usgs.com). The United Nations Office for Coordination of Humanitarian Affairs reports that, "in 2010, about 227,000 people were killed due to earthquakes, with over 222,570 from the magnitude 7.0 Haiti event."

An earthquake is a tremendous release of seismic energy in a series of elastic waves and violent tremors in the crust of the earth. The tectonic plates that make up this outermost layer of the earth are loose fragments of land. They form the continents and the ocean basin. Over decades or centuries, tectonic pressures force the plates to move. Stresses accumulate as the plates move, collide, and slide past or over each other. When the built up energy can no longer be contained it suddenly snaps and releases as a tectonic earthquake.

An earthquake is the most dramatic and far-reaching of natural disasters with its runaway freight train roar, shaking ground, and powerful shock waves. The destruction is magnified when the earthquake hits an urban area collapsing buildings, fracturing freeways, exploding gas lines, and igniting fires. Downed power lines and electric grid lockups can trigger massive power outages and blackouts; shutting down cities and transportation systems. Other disasters can follow or accompany an earthquake, extending the already significant devastation. Gigantic ocean waves called tsunamis can be set off by the seismic activity and power into distant coastlines at rocket speed. Floods, volcanic eruptions, and landslides can either be spawned by an earthquake or strike simultaneously. Earthquakes can also be created by volcanic eruptions on land or in the ocean. Examples of man-made earthquakes include underground mine collapses and nuclear explosions.

The bounds of earthquake country are expanding. The New Madrid Fault Earthquake Zone is *six times larger* than the Pacific Coast's San Andreas Fault and it lies in the middle of the United States, affecting seven states. Geologists and scientists have amassed huge amounts of data on all aspects of earthquakes. However, even with 21st century technology and equipment, they remain unable to predict these seismic events in specific time frames. The expectation, based on all scientists know now, is that those living in earthquake country should be ready for a big event within their lifetime. Because of the magnitude of destruction and havoc these disasters cause, proactively taking steps to ensure

Earthquakes

survival makes good common sense. To have even more information, you can install an application on your smart phone, iPad, or tablet that will alert you to earthquake activity. See the Resource Guide at the back of the book for further details.

Below are very specific steps to take to protect you and your household before, during, and after an earthquake.

Before the Quake

Outside
- ❑ Check power line locations so you know what areas to avoid.
- ❑ Remove weak or diseased tree limbs that might damage power lines.
- ❑ Hire an arborist to remove trees that might fall on the house.
- ❑ Check with neighbors on unsafe or diseased trees near your property.
- ❑ Brace chimney, masonry, concrete walls, and foundations.
- ❑ Check on land use and seismic codes before building or remodeling.
- ❑ Secure frame of picture windows with plywood, if possible.
- ❑ Anchor porches and decks to the main house.
- ❑ Upgrade to meet current building and seismic codes as necessary.
- ❑ Practice turning off water at the street main.
- ❑ Check gas meter, place tool nearby—in the emergency kit or with a neighbor.
- ❑ Check if seismic shutoff valves are used by your local gas company.

Interior Hazards
- Brace ceiling joists under chimney with plywood.
- Bolt floor joists to the foundation with anchor bolts or steel plates.
- Bolt stories together, reinforce joints.
- Brace inside of wall between foundation and first floor with sheathing.
- Shore up garage with exposed studs with a half inch of plywood.
- Sheath around picture windows.
- Check fuse box and replace bad fuses, stock spares.
- Have a licensed electrician upgrade fuse boxes to circuit breakers.
- Check circuit breaker boxes for loose or worn out breakers, and replace.
- Hire a licensed electrician to upgrade circuit breakers to current code.
- Call a retrofitting company for quotes on this type of work.

Inside the House
- Get insurance, and inventory your possessions and valuables.
- Build an emergency kit; store food, water, and supplies.
- Make up satellite emergency kits for bedrooms, work, school, and car.
- Pick a safe place away from the house to reunite afterwards.
- Establish a message center where household members can leave notes.
- Find closets and safe places away from flying objects or glass in each room.
- Practice drop, cover, and hold on tight (www.redcross.org).

Earthquakes   *137*

- ❏ Store flammables, paint, and pesticides in locked cabinets on low shelves.
- ❏ Keep toxic chemicals in outside sheds with securely latched doors.
- ❏ Bolt water heater to wall with safety straps or cables.
- ❏ Bolt down gas appliances with safety cables or straps.
- ❏ Lock rollers on large appliances, kitchen racks or islands.
- ❏ Strap plumbing and gas lines to walls, ceilings, or floors every two feet.
- ❏ Put flexible hoses on gas appliances.
- ❏ Room by room, secure and bolt heavy furniture.
- ❏ Contain TV's in securely latched cabinets, bolt flat screen TV's to walls.
- ❏ Brace overhead light fixtures.
- ❏ Move heavy items and mirrors away from sitting and sleeping areas.
- ❏ Apply safety film to glass doors and windows.
- ❏ Get training in first aid and CPR.
- ❏ Take classes in fire safety, practice fire extinguisher operation and fire drills.
- ❏ Network locally by attending community and neighborhood meetings.

During the Quake

Outdoors
- ✓ If walking outdoors, stay outdoors and don't panic.
- ✓ Avoid trees, power lines, tall buildings, streetlights, and overpasses.
- ✓ Do not go near or pick up a downed power line.
- ✓ Look for an open meadow and go there.
- ✓ Do not seek shelter in a damaged building.

- ✓ Near mountains, slopes, or cliffs, watch out for falling rocks or avalanches.
- ✓ If driving on a bridge or overpass, pull over slowly, park in a clear spot.
  - Stay in the car with seat belt on and wait for help.
- ✓ Never park under a bridge, overpass or by a roadway sign that could fall.
- ✓ If power lines fall on your car, close windows, stay put, wait for help.
- ✓ If near a bay, lake, or river, quickly head for high ground.
- ✓ If at the coast, heed tsunami sirens, leave the beach, and go to high ground.
- ✓ Listen to the radio for updates on conditions; follow official instructions.
- ✓ Drive cautiously to avoid roadside hazards when returning home.
- ✓ Be aware that traffic signals may not work.

Indoors
- ✓ If in bed, curl up, hang on tight, and pull a pillow over your head.
- ✓ If in bed, hold on to the bed frame or roll onto floor and take cover.
- ✓ Wait for the shaking to stop before finding pets or rescuing others.
- ✓ Move away from brick, glass doors, windows, skylights, and mirrors.
- ✓ Move away from large pieces of furniture.
- ✓ Get into a closet away from flying objects and glass, and secure door.
- ✓ Duck under a desk or sturdy table and hang on tight until the shaking stops.

Earthquakes

- ✓ If in a wheelchair, go to an inside wall away from falling glass and objects.
  - Set the brake, cover your head, hang on tight, and stay put.
- ✓ In a crowded theater or auditorium, stay seated, duck, cover, and hold on.
- ✓ Be aware that fire alarms and sprinklers may go off without a fire present.
- ✓ In a high-rise building, take the stairs, not elevators.
- ✓ In any public building use emergency exits.
- ✓ If at work, duck, cover, and hold on tight.
- ✓ Stay away from windows and masonry.

After the Quake

Indoors
- ❑ If you are injured, administer first aid, check in with others next.
- ❑ If trapped under debris, cover your mouth with a cloth or shirtsleeve.
  - Stay still, do not light a match.
  - Be aware that shouting can lead to inhalation of toxic fumes.
  - Find a pipe or object to tap on to signal rescuers.
- ❑ Dress everyone in protective pants, shirts, heavy shoes, and gloves.
- ❑ Assist others and render first aid as safety permits.
- ❑ Put out small fires with fire extinguisher or evacuate the house.
- ❑ Tune into crank or battery radio for news and official instructions.
- ❑ Check your mobile device for emergency alerts and notifications.

- ❑ Quickly assess any hazards inside.
- ❑ Be aware that a rotten egg smell signals a gas leak; do not light a match.
- ❑ Turn gas off at meter with wrench or shutoff tool.
- ❑ Do not turn on light switches or garage door openers in case of gas leaks.
- ❑ Use manual override on garage door to exit.
- ❑ Check for water leaks and flooding.
- ❑ Evacuate in case of flood.
- ❑ Shut all toilet lids in case of sewer backup.
- ❑ Use portable toilets stored with camping supplies.
- ❑ Plug drains in tubs, showers, and sinks to block sewer backup.
- ❑ Check for loose or broken wires or shorts, but do not touch wires.
- ❑ If electrical damage is found, shut off power at the circuit breaker box.
- ❑ Check for structural damage: walls, floors, stairways, doors, and windows.
- ❑ Check furnace, evacuate if ducts or pipes are torn exposing asbestos.
- ❑ Clean up toxic chemical spills, inflammables, and glass.
- ❑ Do not eat food found near broken glass.
- ❑ Turn off and unplug all damaged appliances.
- ❑ Put landline phones back on hooks, check for dial tone.
- ❑ Do not use the phone to call 9-1-1, except for life or death emergencies.
- ❑ Check cell phone reception and call out-of-area contact.
- ❑ To get emergency drinking water, thaw refrigerator ice cubes.
  - Get non-chemically treated water from a toilet tank, not from bowl.

Earthquakes

- ▪ Take water from hot water heater, purify with bleach using eyedropper.
- ☐ Take down unsecured pictures and artwork; leave fallen objects down.
- ☐ Prepare for aftershocks and possible evacuation.
- ☐ Wrap breakables in blankets.
- ☐ Open cabinets, closets carefully to avoid falling objects and broken dishes.
- ☐ Post a handwritten sign on your front door for rescuers to see if you are "OK" or if you "Need Help."
- ☐ Stay in the house only if it is safe to do so.
- ☐ Follow evacuation instructions from authorities.
- ☐ If leaving home, provide your destination in your designated message center.

Outdoors

- ☐ If trapped under debris, cover your mouth with a cloth or shirtsleeve.
  - ▪ Stay still, do not light a match and do not call out; avoid inhaling toxic dust.
  - ▪ Find a pipe or object to tap on to signal rescuers.
- ☐ Check the house for chimney damage; remove loose bricks from roof.
- ☐ Clear fallen bricks and broken glass from pathways.
- ☐ Check for separation of exterior walls, attachments, porches, and decks.
- ☐ Turn off street water main in case of broken sewer line(s).
- ☐ Use duct tape and plastic sheeting to mend cracked windows.
- ☐ Use plywood to board up broken or blown out windows.
- ☐ If the gas is turned off, do not relight the pilot; call the gas company.

- ❏ Evacuate if gas smell persists or if explosion occurs.
  - Evacuate if fire breaks out.
  - Evacuate if mudslide or landslide occurs.
  - Evacuate if flooding arises.
- ❏ Go to high ground in case of tsunami warnings.

Away from Home and Returning Home
- ❏ Stay where you are until the shaking stops.
- ❏ If you are alone and injured, treat injuries from your first aid kit.
- ❏ If you are with others, check on them next and administer first aid.
- ❏ If trapped under debris, cover your mouth with a cloth or shirtsleeve.
  - Stay still to avoid inhaling toxic dust; do not light a match.
  - Find a pipe or object to tap on to signal rescuers.
- ❏ Check radio reports on road safety conditions before driving or walking.
- ❏ If you must abandon your car, park away from overpasses and road signs.
- ❏ Do not park near tall buildings, trees, and power lines.
- ❏ Do not go into any structure where the roof or walls have collapsed.
- ❏ Use your cell phone to call, text, or email your out-of-area contact person.
- ❏ If you can't get home, use safe routes to go to your meeting spot.
- ❏ Upon returning home, do not go inside if the house appears at all unstable.
- ❏ If the ground is shifting, do not go inside; evacuate instead.

Earthquakes

- ❑ If the house is stable and the gas is off, do not turn it back on yourself.
  - Call the gas company to relight the pilot on the gas meter.
- ❑ Heed tsunami warnings and move away from the beach to higher ground.
- ❑ Evacuate in case of a flood.
- ❑ Evacuate in the event of landslides.
- ❑ Expect aftershocks for 24 hours, days, weeks, or months later.
- ❑ Restock your emergency supplies; be ready for aftershocks.

LANDSLIDES

Landslides are mighty forces of nature that harness gravity to pull great masses of earth downward, and they can strike as disasters anytime and anywhere in the world. Tonnages of soil, mud, boulders, and debris plummet down hills, cliffs, and mountains far and wide; often happening in the blink of an eye. The velocity of landslide flows has been clocked at 50 to 200-mph, and slow creeping movement can also develop quietly and gradually over years or decades of time. For live action views of landslides, check out the videos posted online (http://video.nationalgeographic.com/video/player/environment/environment-natural-disasters/landslides-and-more/landslides.html).

Certain physical locations on hillsides and near cliffs or canyons are more susceptible to slides, slumps, spreads, rock falls, and mudflows than others, while steep slopes of over 10 to 15 degrees are especially vulnerable. Changing seasonal conditions are documented to optimize risks for earth movement as well. Hot weather that dries up forests and brush sets the scene for summer wildfires that burn off slope stabilizing vegetation. Wet seasons with prolonged or heavy downpours or sudden flash floods loosen soil and mud, propelling it downward. Gushing underground springs have also displaced earth and excess water from rapid snowmelt has perpetuated flooding, mountain rockslides, and avalanches.

In the warm spring of 1983, melting snow saturated the mountain slope near Thistle, Utah. It led to a mile-long flow of mud and debris that dammed up the Spanish Fork River creating a 160-foot deep lake that flooded out the entire town. The slide destroyed the railroad tracks and cut off travel between Salt Lake City and Denver. With a cost of $200 million the event was declared a disaster by United States President Ronald Reagan. Land movement has continued over the decades, and residents have been unable to return home.

Numerous natural disasters have moved the earth and spawned landslides that have triggered other disasters, and potent earthquakes have rocked and rolled the land sweeping away tons of loose terra firma in mere seconds. In 1958, a magnitude 7.9 quake struck along the Fair Weather Fault in the Alaska Panhandle plunging 40 million cubic yards of glacier rock 3,000 feet down into Gilbert Inlet. The submarine impact spurred a tsunami wave that scaled the cliff and crested at a record height of 1,720 feet. In 1980, the biggest landslide in world history sprang from the volcanic eruption of Mount St. Helens in Washington's Cascade Mountains in the United States.

Man-made disasters bring on deadly landslides as well. Improper landscape maintenance and construction has been shown to imperil the natural terrain, property and structures, and it has also threatened neighborhood and community populations. Water can be a viable force. Overflowing sprinklers and irrigation systems have deterred slope stability, eroded hillsides and ultimately caused slopes to fail, tumbling land masses, buildings, and homes down in destructive slides. Leaking plumbing, broken sewer lines, disconnected downspouts, and lack of storm drain control can change groundwater with the same end result.

Removal of vegetation or trees and their important tap root systems can invite erosion of slopes and set the stage for earth movement. Installation of new retaining walls, additions of heavy rock or hardscape to the top of slopes, removal of existing retaining walls, and subtraction of material from the bottom of a slope can all be detrimental to the stability of the terrain. Construction of any kind on the topside of slopes, hillsides, cliffs, or canyons can put structures and their occupants at great risk. Entire coastal subdivisions built on oceanfront dune lands have collapsed when their foundations were destroyed by the naturally shifting sands and soils they were built on.

In the United Kingdom in 2008, the fossil rich 95-mile long stretch of the Jurassic Coast was the site of the worst landslide in a century. Chunks of land the size of automobiles cascaded down the high cliffs of Dorsett and fell into the sea and onto the beach. The priceless fossils date back 185 million years, and are considered a national treasure. Speculations on the cause of the disaster cited erosion from global warming's climate change, but it has remained unproven. For a more detailed description of landslides and mud flows, go online (www.bt.cdc.gov/disasters/landslides.asp).

In August 2010, the drama of a man-made landslide made news worldwide. An unstable gold and copper mine collapsed in San Jose, Chile and entombed 33 miners. For years, the men had risked their lives to do their jobs, and now they waited to be saved. The world waited too, for a spellbinding 69 days. The underground entrapment was the longest one on record, and the miraculous survival and rescue of the miners united people everywhere. The cost of the rescue alone was a reported $22 million. Psychiatrists who examined the men cautioned that additional costs could lie ahead for the survivors in terms of their ability to live normal lives.

Preparation is clearly needed for any type of landslide. Below is an outline of how to handle a landslide.

Before the Landslide

- ❑ Be aware that landslides have struck in all 50 of the United States and worldwide.
- ❑ Know that landslides hit without warning.
- ❑ Hire a geologist to analyze soil stability before buying a home.
- ❑ Be aware that houses on top of slopes or hills are at risk.

- ❑ Be aware that houses near cliffs and canyons can experience landslides.
- ❑ Get homeowner's or renter's insurance and inventory possessions.
- ❑ Check with your insurance agent for landslide coverage.
- ❑ Be aware that expanded coverage will carry an additional premium.
- ❑ Check drainage of your property and manage water flow.
- ❑ Note the irrigation and vegetation of uphill neighbors.
- ❑ Replant any uphill areas where fire has burned off vegetation.
- ❑ Install drain fields or French drains as needed to divert water.
- ❑ Dig trenches to direct water away from the house.
- ❑ Keep gutters and downspouts clear.
- ❑ Clean out catch basins and drains.
- ❑ Manage storm water run-off and monitor neighbors' run-off.
- ❑ Install flexible pipes to avoid gas and water leaks.
- ❑ Ask local nurseries about planting deep root plants that are native to your area for better ground stability.
- ❑ Plant fast growing trees with long tap roots for steep slopes.
- ❑ Build retaining walls on slopes upon the advice of geotechnical engineers.
- ❑ Terrace steep slopes with the help of a civil engineer consultant.
- ❑ Minimize irrigation systems on slopes and control and monitor water flow.
- ❑ Do not remove anything from the base of a slope; consult a civil engineer.
- ❑ Consult a civil engineer before adding rock or other materials to slope top.

Landslides

- ☐ Contact a plumbing contractor to inspect sewer cracks or breaks.

During the Landslide

- ✓ If you hear water running, check property for broken pipes.
- ✓ Check for any present dangers.
- ✓ Evacuate if any of the following conditions occur:
  - Rumbling that gets louder.
  - House creaks or unusual noises.
  - Boulders crash on the slope.
  - Trees breaking or cracking.
  - Floors or walls tilting.
  - Cracks appearing in the house.
  - Cracks opening in the ground.
  - Water pooling in drains, on the ground or stops moving.
  - Porches and decks separate from the house.
  - If you suspect you are in any eminent danger.

After the Landslide

- ☐ Only return home once the area has been certified safe by authorities.
- ☐ Inspect driveways, foundation, and retaining walls for cracks.
- ☐ Check for trees that are bowed or leaning.
- ☐ Check for new cracks on stucco, plaster, or brick exterior of the house.
- ☐ Look for bulging in your surrounding landscape and concrete walks.
- ☐ Look for cracks in the road, sidewalk, or pathways that are widening.
- ☐ Check for tilted fences, utility poles, and trees.

- ❑ See if porches or decks have pulled away from structures or supports.
- ❑ Check at the base of the slope for any bulges in the ground.
- ❑ Inspect the ground for water breaking through in new areas.
- ❑ Check chimneys for cracks or visually inspect them for tilting.
- ❑ Clean up loose bricks on pathways.
- ❑ Avoid areas where soil has parted.

Inside

- ❑ Do not go into your house if the ground is unstable.
- ❑ Only go in the house if it is safe and not tilted or unstable.
- ❑ Inspect interior walls and floors for tilting and cracks.
- ❑ Check doors and windows to see if they open and close properly.
- ❑ Be aware sticking windows and doors may indicate instability of slow creeping land. Have an inspection by a contractor.
- ❑ Check for plumbing and gas line leaks before using utilities, and avoid striking matches or smoking for hours after an incident.

Outside

- ❑ Call utility provider to turn the gas back on.
- ❑ If gas smell does not dissipate after opening windows, evacuate.
- ❑ Check on tilted trees, fences, and buildings that could come down later.
- ❑ Report downed utility lines to authorities.
- ❑ Listen for emergency information on news sites or via a mobile device.

TSUNAMIS

Literally translated, the word tsunami means harbor wave, but in reality tsunamis originate hundreds of miles away from their coastal destination points in the region known as the Ring of Fire in the Pacific Ocean's distant depths. Ruptures and fault line fractures in the huge continental plates below the ocean floor propel seismic eruptions, and earthquakes power giant tsunami sea waves at breakneck speeds of up to 600-mph. Submarine avalanches, landslides, and volcanic eruptions can also drive tsunami forces inland and send them rocketing through the water to their ports of culmination. On top of the open ocean, the wide span between wave crests of 100 miles or more makes the turbulent tsunami action barely noticeable, but as the water turns shallow near shore, the mighty waves arrive in a fanfare with high-rise surges of up to 200 feet. The water topples onto shore, pounding coastlines and swamping harbors and bays. The force races inland, plowing up cities and landscapes and depleting energy by crashing back and forth in narrow river inlets.

The island nation of Japan has suffered the greatest number of tsunamis in the world, and on March 11, 2011 the news media held the stunned world witness to epic destruction. A three-fold disaster rocked and battered the country's eastern coast. It began with a magnitude 9.0 earthquake that jet streamed a 30-foot high tsunami resulting in a wall of water powering onto shore with wrecking ball force. It lifted city buildings and houses in one fell swoop, downing power everywhere. The Fukushima Daiichi nuclear power plant was hit, shutting down the reactors' cooling system and enabling a meltdown and radioactive release. The tsunami traveled three miles inland ravaging everything in its wake. The current death count is 24,000 and expected to rise. More than 90,000 people are living in shelters. From this occurrence, tsunami warnings went out to 50 countries over the Pacific from Japan to the west coast of the United States.

The Pacific Ring of Fire has always been the most active staging ground for earthquakes, volcanic eruptions, and tsunamis. In 2004, a mammoth 9.1 magnitude earthquake in the Indian Ocean generated a tsunami that spread turmoil and devastation to 13 countries including Indonesia, Sri Lanka, India, and Thailand with a quarter of a million killed. In 2010 Sumatra, Indonesia was the site of a 7.7 magnitude submarine quake that triggered a tsunami from 13 miles under the ocean floor and swept away 10 villages near the Mentawai Islands. One hundred and eight inhabitants died. In the same year, on the heels of a volcanic eruption, a tsunami caused thousands to be evacuated near central Java, badly damaging the Islands of Mentawai, South Pagai and North Pagai. There was no warning system available, which worsened the disaster's impact.

The world record for the highest tsunami wave was set in the United States during the summer of 1958 in Alaska's Panhandle, and topped 1,720 feet. According to the USGS, the precursor to the tsunami was an earthquake that broke out on the Fairweather Fault in Lituya Bay. The quake launched a landslide and 40 million cubic yards of glacier rock plunged 3,000 feet down into the bay. The thunderous impact spurred a tsunami that rose up the cliff face, shearing off all the timber and sinking two boats.

Tsunamis are huge, powerful forces of nature often triggered by other disasters. They can cause enormous damage and loss of life. Tsunamis have been shown to beget other disasters including man-made disasters like Japan's nuclear power plant meltdown. Tsunamis are monitored at the Pacific Tsunami Warning Center (www.weather.gov/ptwc).

The following are action steps to take before, during, and after a tsunami occurs.

Before the Tsunami

Outside
- Drive or walk prearranged evacuation routes.
- Watch the ocean for sudden low tide and exposure of the ocean floor.
- Be aware of trembling ground rolling up and down in waves.
- If you are in a boat at sea, stay at sea. Far from shore, you may only notice a slight rise in the water.
- If you are in a boat or ship near shore, put it out to sea if a warning comes.
- Monitor news feeds and tsunami alert warnings and evacuation instructions.
- Know that if a tsunami watch is issued, an earthquake has been detected under the sea and a tsunami might occur.
- Go to high ground, even a cliff over the ocean, and wait for further bulletins.
- If you hear sirens or other warning signals, evacuate as trained.
- Do not approach the ocean. Always seek the highest ground you can.
- If you are in a bay or river inlet, be aware that tsunamis can grow very tall and dangerous in shallow water.
- Stay away from buildings that could topple.
- Stay away from bridges and other structures that could be washed away.

Inside
- ❏ Get insurance and inventory your possessions.
- ❏ Attend first aid and CPR classes.
- ❏ Attend neighborhood and community meetings.
- ❏ Store emergency supplies where you can get to them in a hurry.
- ❏ Secure your home.
- ❏ Plan household, family, and neighborhood check-in methods for after the disaster.
- ❏ Determine a good source for monitoring tsunami warnings and evacuation instructions via radio, cell phone, or Internet.
- ❏ Prepare to go to high ground and wait for further bulletins.

During the Tsunami
- ✓ Avoid bridges that could wash away.
- ✓ Remain calm and wait for news and instruction.
- ✓ Contain dogs on leashes, cats in carriers.
- ✓ If you are in a boat—know not to come ashore, wait until the all clear sign has been given.
- ✓ Wait for the all-clear sirens or signal to return home.

After the Tsunami
- ❏ Check for injuries and render first aid.
- ❏ Do not return home until advised by authorities and given the all clear signal.
- ❏ Check your home's exterior for chimney damage, separation of exterior walls, attachments, and damage to porches and decks.
- ❏ Do not go inside the house if it looks unstable.
- ❏ Follow your emergency plan.

Tsunamis

- ❏ Use your out-of-area contact person to relay messages.
- ❏ Check Google and Red Cross sites online for information locating missing individuals.
- ❏ Have a licensed inspector evaluate your home for safety.
- ❏ Approach animals with caution; contain your pets.

VOLCANIC ERUPTIONS

Volcanic eruptions are often launched in The Ring of Fire in the Pacific Ocean where seismic powered earthquakes and tsunamis are prevalent. Volcanoes have erupted in the countries of Japan, New Zealand, Iceland, Ecuador, Costa Rica, the West Indies, Italy, and the United States in Kilauea, on the Big Island of Hawaii—one of the most active volcanoes on earth. It began to erupt in 1983 and continues on in present day where it attracts scientific study from volcanologists coming from all over the world. Elsewhere in the galaxy Mars, Neptune, and Jupiter all host volcanoes.

Back on Earth in Iceland, the volcano Eyjafjallajokull erupted in 2010 and triggered the biggest lava flow in 10,000 years; ejecting a vast cloud of ash into the atmosphere, grounding European airline traffic for a week. The massive shut down was the largest since WWII, and 10 million air travelers were disrupted. A year later, another Icelandic volcano erupted with its biggest blast in 100 years. Grimsvotn, the country's second largest volcano, blew a 12-mile high plume of ash towards Scotland and the continent of Europe, and led to the closure of Iceland's International Airport and the cancellation of flights by British Airways and other European carriers. Fears that the previous year's air traffic troubles would recur were on the rise, but the Iceland Meteorological Office downplayed the concerns.

The riveting drama of the volcano's fiery explosion starts with seismic turbulence in the center of the earth. Fifteen major pieces of the earth's crust, called plates, float on the hot molten layer under the surface (known as magma), much like pieces of crackers in a bowl of soup. A volcanic eruption is often created from two plates rubbing up against one another and overlapping in piggyback fashion, with one plate plunged deep into the earth 50 to 60 miles below the surface of the crust. The atmosphere there has been compared to a giant nuclear power plant, fueled by the breakdown of radioactive elements. When the plummeting plate shatters and melts, its enormous velocity sends pieces of rock propelling up through the cracks in the earth's surface to burst forth from the crater.

The eruption releases a gigantic cloud of gas and molten lava flows like a river onto the terrain below. When the lava hardens to rock, it forms mountains, prairies, coastlines, and offshore islands. Volcanic eruptions can also be touched off by earthquakes that originate in the middle of a plate. Volcanoes worldwide have been tracked for over three decades by the Smithsonian Natural Museum of Natural History. The findings can be seen online (www.volcano.si.edu/world).

Below are detailed steps for dealing with a volcanic disaster.

Before the Eruption

Outside
- If building a house in a lava zone, consider building with fire-retardant materials.
- Build with fire-resistant treated wood products and aluminum.
- Plant trees and bushes sparsely to avoid a path of fuel for a lava flow fire.
- Tear off wood shake roof and replace with noncombustible roof.
- Use asphalt shingles, tile, slate, cement, sheet metal, or aluminum roofing materials.
- Trim trees and shrubs away from roofs of your home, garage, or shop.

Volcanic Eruptions

- ❏ Plant large trees a minimum of 10 feet from your home's exterior.
- ❏ Water and prune the landscaping well to create a protective fire line.
- ❏ Keep tree branches clear of power lines.
- ❏ Call the utility company if nearby trees are touching wires.
- ❏ Haul away yard debris before it piles up and becomes a fire hazard.
- ❏ Maintain a 30-foot defensible space firebreak around your home. Eliminate any combustible vegetation.
- ❏ If you live on a hillside or a forest, clear a perimeter of 100 feet or more as a firebreak.
- ❏ Clean gutters and roof regularly to remove combustible leaves and needles.
- ❏ Follow local burning safety restrictions when disposing of debris.
- ❏ Store all flammables away from the house.
- ❏ Stack firewood away from the house; stack on a flat surface, be aware fires can travel uphill.
- ❏ Have an adequate water supply to fight fires in rural areas.
- ❏ Fill water tanks, cisterns, fire hydrants, or wells and test with high volume pumps.
- ❏ Store cars and machinery inside to protect engines from ash.
- ❏ Maintain swimming pools, ponds, or storage tanks. Keep portable pumps in working order.
- ❏ In case of electrical failure, have an alternate power backup system like a generator for well pumps.
- ❏ Test water hoses for leaks and make sure they are long enough to reach all around the exterior of your home.

- ❏ Keep a hose with a nozzle attachment connected to an outside outlet.
- ❏ Have a ladder tall enough to reach your roof.
- ❏ Stock firefighting tools: an axe, rake, chainsaw, a long-handled, round-point shovel, and a two-and-a-half gallon water bucket.
- ❏ For emergency and fire truck access, maintain two-way roads with parking lanes.
- ❏ Build roads that slope less than 10 feet per 100 feet for accessibility of emergency vehicles.
- ❏ Clear from the roadway flammable brush 60 feet wide along the right of way to prevent a wildfire hazard.
- ❏ Be aware that no man-made effort can stop molten rock.

Inside
- ❏ Get insurance and inventory your possessions.
  - Secure this information where you can retrieve it in case you file a claim.
- ❏ Attend community meetings on volcanoes, earthquakes, and emergency evacuation procedures.
- ❏ Take Red Cross first aid, CPR, and fire safety classes.
- ❏ Call a household meeting and create a plan of where to meet if separated and what to do about pets and livestock.
- ❏ Plan escape routes—one by foot and two by car.
- ❏ Map your routes and send to your out-of-area contact person. Know how to access these maps by mobile device.
- ❏ Synch up your escape routes for each household member by phone or Internet.
- ❏ Store emergency supplies, food, and water.
- ❏ Store disposable dust masks to protect against inhaling volcanic ash.
- ❏ Post by every phone the number to call in case of a fire.

Volcanic Eruptions

- ❏ Install portable smoke detectors outside every sleeping area, on every level of your home, in your garage and in other buildings on your property.
- ❏ Use button to test smoke alarms twice a year.
- ❏ Keep extra smoke alarm batteries on hand for replacements.
- ❏ Keep ABC fire extinguishers in the kitchen and hallways, test and replace immediately if faulty.
- ❏ Conduct fire drills, including walking and driving evacuation routes and practice them throughout the year.
- ❏ Draw a floor plan, find two ways to exit from every room, and conduct drills.
- ❏ Get rope or chain ladders for upstairs rooms and practice using in drills.

During the Eruption

- ✓ Turn off gas at the meter to avoid explosion(s).
- ✓ Close doors, windows, and fireplace dampers.
- ✓ Put on heavy shoes and protective clothing.
- ✓ Secure animals and livestock in closed shelters.
- ✓ Take your stored supplies and complete evacuation procedures.
- ✓ Tune into phone alerts or news feeds for updates on the volcano.
- ✓ Do not return home until the eruption is declared over, and the lava flow and fires have stopped.
- ✓ Prepare to travel on a route confirmed to be safe.
- ✓ Stay upwind and upstream of the volcano.
- ✓ If driving, use extreme caution. Take only confirmed routes.
  - Abandon your car if lava and fire encroaches, and take a route away from the fire.

After the Eruption

- ❑ Assist others and render first aid as safety permits.
- ❑ Wear your disposable dust masks to avoid respiratory irritation.
- ❑ Check radio and social media reports for confirmed information and instructions.
- ❑ Check on tsunami warnings and go to high ground if evacuation is necessary.
- ❑ Be aware that earthquake aftershocks can occur after an eruption.
- ❑ Check on location of Red Cross Disaster Stations, shelters, and animal holding areas.
- ❑ Use caution going home. Do not return unless advised by authorities that conditions are safe and roads are clear.
- ❑ If driving is necessary, drive with caution.
- ❑ Be aware visibility may be very poor if it is raining volcanic ash.
- ❑ Know that mudslides and landslides can also occur.
- ❑ Avoid volcano damaged areas and lava flow areas.
- ❑ Know where your neighborhood or community emergency staging area will be located.
- ❑ Check your home's exterior for damage and stability. If an earthquake has occurred, use due caution and follow procedures.
- ❑ Do not go inside if it appears unsafe.
- ❑ If other household or family members are not there, call or text your out-of-area contact person.
- ❑ Follow your plan for locating one another and reuniting in a safe place.
- ❑ Approach animals with caution; comfort and contain them as much as possible.
- ❑ Check and repair fenced areas for animals.

- ❏ Beware of loose or dangling electrical wires; do not touch.
- ❏ Check gas appliance connections for signs of gas leaks.
- ❏ Evacuate if you smell gas.
- ❏ Do not light a match.

HURRICANES

Hurricanes are immense and spectacular rotary storms born in the family called tropical cyclones. These turbulent seasonal events arise in the Caribbean Sea and the Atlantic Ocean from June to December, hitting hardest from August to September. The titanic forces of nature can burgeon up to 300 or 400 miles in diameter with pelting, sideways rain, and crushing 75 to 200-mph winds whirling around the calm and eerie center known as the eye of the storm. The driving forces of tropical cyclones have propelled storm surges, tidal waves, floods, landslides, and tornados; multiplying the severity and breadth of calamity. The name "hurricane" can be traced back to the legend of the Mayan god Hurakan who beset hapless mortals with deadly storms and floods. The cyclones have lived up to their destructive reputation wherever they make landfall: be it the tropical regions of the Caribbean Islands, the West Indies, the Canary Islands, or the Gulf of Mexico. Six to eight monster storms exact an annual toll of over $4.9 billion in damages along the eastern and southern coasts of the United States alone.

In 2005, the infamous Hurricane Katrina wrought disaster in three states and became the costliest storm in United States history with estimated losses and impact tipped to $150 billion. According to the National Oceanic Atmospheric Association (NOAA), the storm's driving winds measured 175-mph, and its storm surges rose to 28 feet above normal tide. The wake of destruction spread over 100 miles in Louisiana, Mississippi, and Alabama; and the enormous disaster also spawned a reported 33 tornados. Located six feet below sea level, the city of New Orleans was inundated with flooding when its aging 12-foot levee system was overtopped and breached by the nearly 30-foot high water surge. This natural disaster morphed into a man-made disaster due to the levee's inadequate design, construction, and maintenance. The costs were high. One million Gulf Coast residents lost their homes and were evacuated and re-located and 1,836 people were confirmed dead with an additional 705 residents listed as missing. The economy suffered and hundreds of thousands of workers lost their jobs. Oil and grain exports were down by 18 to 20 percent, and Mississippi's forestry lands lost $5 billion.

Other economically damaging hurricanes have topped the billion-dollar mark as well. The next costliest tropical cyclone on record was Hurricane Andrew in 1992 with almost $27 billion in damages and 26 lives lost. The modest tropical wave that arose on the West African coast migrated between Bermuda and Puerto Rico westward and grew to hurricane status. The storm lambasted the Bahamas and South Florida with 169-mph winds and 17-foot storm surges, and reeled into the Gulf of Mexico touching down in Louisiana where it packed another wallop by unleashing a powerful tornado that twisted through the southeastern part of the state.

In 2004, another powerful tropical cyclone traveled far and wide on a destructive path that spun off over 100 tornados in the southeastern United States. Hurricane Ivan began on the west coast of Africa and pelted the Caribbean with 160-mph winds over Grenada, the Dominican Republic, and Jamaica. The storm tore into Grand Cayman, swamped the island, and wrecked all but five percent of the buildings left standing. It rode the Yucatan channel, battered Cuba and moved to the Gulf of Mexico and the United States; setting off a flurry of tornados and heavy rainfall in the south. The NOAA reported 92 people killed, and the cost reached $14.2 billion—the third largest total on record.

As recent history shows, hurricanes recur annually and

bring a long and checkered legacy of enormous destruction. The toll can be measured in lives lost, property and infrastructure damage, economic costs in the billions, displaced populations, and eroded or obliterated land. In a climate dramatically altered by global warming and rising sea temperatures, meteorologists and other experts have ratcheted up forecasts for greater incidences and severity of storms along coastal regions. NOAA has named the highest probability targets of the storms to Miami; Cape Hatteras, North Carolina; San Juan, Puerto Rico; and New Orleans. The agency has noted that the global risk will grow as a trend to live in coastal regions increases. For information on hurricane preparedness, mitigation, and recovery, see the publications posted on the National Weather Service site in conjunction with the National Hurricane Center (www.nhc.noaa.gov). You can also visit the website for up-to-the-minute hurricane tracking and warnings.

Below are very specific steps to take to protect you and your household before, during, and after a hurricane.

Before the Hurricane

Outside
- ❑ Remove weak or diseased tree branches.
- ❑ Hire a licensed arborist to remove hazardous trees.
- ❑ Check locations of nearby power lines.
- ❑ Work with neighbors to eliminate tree hazards near your properties.
- ❑ Check roof for loose shingles and make repairs.
- ❑ Board up windows, tape glass that can break from flying debris.
- ❑ Know that wind pressure can shatter large windows.
- ❑ Contain pets and livestock.

- Keep your car's gas tank filled with gas in case evacuation is needed.
- Secure garbage cans, lawn furniture, and barbeques in a shed.
- Store gardening tools and lawnmowers in a garage or in secured sheds.
- Move children's toys and objects that could be hurled by the wind.
- If at the beach, watch for approaching waves.
- Leave low-lying areas due to danger from high tides and flooding.
- If swimming or in a boat, get to shore and seek shelter.
- Secure the boat and evacuate to a pre-designated safe area.
- Check your portable radio for news and instructions.

Inside
- Get homeowner's or renter's insurance; inventory your possessions.
- Take first aid and CPR classes.
- Attend community and neighborhood meetings.
- Secure your home room by room.
- Listen for storm advisories and warnings on the radio or TV.
- Check your water, food, first aid supplies, and camping equipment to ensure you have everything you need.
- Move valuables to a floor safe or strong box.
- Check flashlights and portable radio for fresh batteries.
- Fill bathtubs and clean gallon jugs with tap water before contaminated.
- If in a mobile home or RV park, heed storm warnings and go to a designated shelter.

Hurricanes 169

- ❏ Tune in to radio, TV, or public alerts to monitor the storm.
- ❏ Contain pets by leash or carrier.
- ❏ Evacuate according to official instructions.

During the Hurricane

- ✓ If possible, stay inside and wait out the storm.
- ✓ If you have a basement or storm cellar, it is the best place to wait out the storm.
- ✓ If you do not have a basement, go to the lowest floor of your home, away from windows or anything that could cause harm.
- ✓ Do not try to rescue pets or people during the storm.
- ✓ Beware of the eye, the calm center of the storm, as it passes overhead. The calm can last from two minutes to half an hour. Do not leave your shelter until you hear on your emergency radio that the storm has passed.
- ✓ If you are in a wheelchair, set the brake and cover your head.
- ✓ If at work or in public building, follow safety procedures; avoid glass.
- ✓ If walking outside, take cover immediately; get down.
- ✓ If driving, park the car, get out, and seek cover under a freeway overpass, doorway, or stairwell.
- ✓ Avoid power lines, trees, buildings, and windows.
- ✓ Whenever possible, stay calm.

After the Hurricane

- ❏ Avoid driving if possible. If driving is necessary, drive with caution.
- ❏ Know debris may be hazardous and that roads can collapse if undermined.

- ❑ Be aware landslides are also possible after a hurricane.
- ❑ Stay away from riverbanks and streams.
- ❑ Report loose or dangling electrical wires to police or the power company.
- ❑ If separated from your family, call your emergency contact person.
- ❑ Check the outside of the house for damage to chimneys, walls, porches, decks, and stairways.
- ❑ Use caution when returning home or to your designated meeting spot.
- ❑ Do not go into the house if it looks unstable.

Inside
- ❑ Treat yourself first if you are injured.
- ❑ Check others for injuries and render first aid.
- ❑ Put heavy shoes and clothes on everyone.
- ❑ Look for flood warnings, road damage, and emergency routes using your cell phone.
- ❑ Check public alerts or social media for location of shelters.
- ❑ Go to Red Cross disaster stations for emergency medical attention.
- ❑ Check for gas leaks. Do not light a match.
- ❑ Keep animals contained until the situation is under control and the crisis is no longer imminent.
- ❑ Evacuate if directed by authorities.

TORNADOS

Tornados embattle North America, Europe, Asia, West Africa, and regions of the Atlantic carving out half-mile wide paths of destruction with their corkscrew winds flying at speeds of up to 300 miles per hour. Due to their rotating motions, the storms are also known as twisters. The dark funnel clouds are made up of columns of rapidly whirling air, condensation, dust and debris; their shadowy silhouettes emerging against deepening mustard skies in spring and early summer. The high velocity windstorms can be born under the bottom of cumulonimbus clouds or generated in the updraft of thunderstorms or hurricanes moving overhead. In 2001, tropical storm Allison, the deadliest on record, spurred 23 tornados and cost $5 billion and in 2005, Hurricane Katrina followed suit by spinning off 33 twisters.

The grinding roar of a tornado comes from the friction of its high winds against the ground, often likened to a jet plane at takeoff. The sound is a warning of the dangers ahead. The powerful vacuum in the funnel of the storm can seize up and tear apart buildings and houses, scatter rubble everywhere, and demolish entire geographic regions. Everything in the whirlwind's path is threatened.

In North America, the Canadian Prairie Provinces endure a battery of destructive twisters in June, July, and August each year; with more of the speeding funnel clouds churning through the United States than anywhere else in the world. The prevailing hot spot is the central and southeast flatlands of the region named Tornado Alley, and the states of Texas, Arkansas, Oklahoma, Kansas, Nebraska, and Missouri have been annual targets for treacherous strikes. In 2011, the weather pattern La Nina primed the southwest with warm and humid air, and monumentally increased rotary storm activity into a second twister prone region called Dixie

Alley—spreading from the hilly lower Mississippi valley to the tree covered upper Tennessee valley.

In late April and early May of 2011, a militia of tornados hit six southern states in the worst natural disaster since Hurricane Katrina. On April 27, 2011 a 24-hour siege of 312 twisters battered parts of Arkansas, Mississippi, Louisiana, Alabama, Georgia, and Florida. According to the National Weather Service, the tornados set a record for a single storm system. The torque of the whirlwinds ripped trees up by their roots, tore down power lines, splintered homes into kindling, leveled barns, buildings and businesses, and left communities in tatters.

The tornados raged on in the month of May, lambasting terrain and towns with devastation. Dwellers were injured and killed, and mobile home parks were hardest hit. Three hundred and sixty-one deaths were confirmed by *Reuters*. More prolific reports came through via YouTube where storm chaser videos were posted. Alabama Governor Robert Bentley appeared on *Good Morning America*, stating that the death toll was expected to grow, while thousands of families were left homeless. Tornados stretched from Joplin, Missouri to Springfield, Michigan in a day. A social media site was established to deliver resources for disaster affected residents within 48 hours. It directed those who have a need and those who could give help via electronic messaging online (http://rebuildjoplin.org).

Everyday citizens did their best to survive. One Trenton, Georgia salon owner jumped into a tanning bed with her two daughters, hanging on for dear life. The three had survived a twister before by hunkering down in a bathtub, and as veterans of that disaster, they planned to take shelter in the tanning bed before the storm broke. When the tornado plowed into the town of Alberta, Alabama diners at the

Full Moon BBQ ran with waitresses and cooks to safety by ducking into the restaurant's cooler. In Tuscaloosa, two University of Alabama roommates took refuge in a storm cellar, but the house blew away. One was grazed in the head by an airborne jeep and they crawled under the car for cover when it landed. The story made headlines in the campus paper, *The Crimson White*. A bedroom wall was sucked out by the high wind vacuum in Griffin, Georgia, and a sleeping girl was hurled onto her front lawn—mattress and all. Her frantic parents scooped her up and darted into the master bedroom's walk-in closet with two other children in tow.

Fortunately, the emergency response was swift. The Red Cross marshaled a force of 3,700 volunteers, and they sped to the disaster scene. At the Federal level, emergency aid was granted by President Barak Obama, with 1,400 National Guard troops deployed for search and rescue operations. Emergency Food Hotlines were set up with links to food banks to feed the hungry. Several big corporations stepped up with generous assistance. Deluxe Business Services donated $25,000 to the Red Cross, and offered aid to imperiled small businesses. Replacement checks and shipping were free, and business support services included networking, payroll, logo design, web design, and web hosting. The storage giant U-Haul gave away 30 days of free storage, free boxes, and free portable storage to all those impacted. The overall attitude of residents was expressed by Sheriff Patrick Gannon of Trenton, Georgia who said his fellow community members were all thankful to be alive and would come together to rebuild.

Go online to view worldwide areas where tornados frequently strike (www.ncdc.noaa.gov/oa/climate/severe weather/tornadoes.html). A recommended learning tool about tornados can be found online (www.windows2universe.org/earth/Atmosphere/tornado/alley.html).

Below are very specific steps to take to protect you and your household before, during, and after a tornado.

Before the Tornado

Outside
- Fill your car's gas tank.
- Watch the weather; look for darkening skies, stay alert.
- If at the beach, watch for waves coming inland.
- Leave low-lying areas due to danger from high tides and flooding.
- Check your car radio, mobile device, or social media for news and instructions.
- If swimming or in a boat, get to shore and seek shelter.
- Secure the boat or evacuate to a pre-designated safe area.
- Secure or take inside garbage cans, lawn furniture, gardening tools, barbecues, children's toys, and any object the wind could hurl.
- Board up windows, close shutters, and tape glass.
- Be aware that flying debris can shatter big windows and small glass panes.
- Contain pets and livestock.

Inside
- Get insurance and inventory your possessions.
  - Secure this information where you can retrieve it if you file a claim.
- Attend neighborhood and community meetings.
- Take first aid and CPR classes.
- Listen for storm advisories and warnings on the radio or TV.

Tornados

- ❏ Check your emergency supplies and your camping equipment.
- ❏ Move to the side of the house away from the wind.
- ❏ Check flashlights, gather portable radio, fresh batteries, and cell phone hand crank chargers.
- ❏ Fill clean containers, jugs, pans, and even the bathtub before contamination (possible once tornado hits).
- ❏ If you are in a mobile home or RV park, leave as soon as you hear the storm warning and go to a designated shelter.
- ❏ Monitor the storm by listening to the radio, TV, public alerts, or Internet.
- ❏ Prepare to evacuate and follow official's instructions.

During the Tornado

- ✓ If you have a storm cellar, wait out the storm there.
- ✓ If your home is secure, stay in, remain calm, and wait out the storm.
- ✓ Get away from upper floors and open areas, duck into interior hallways, reinforced rooms.
- ✓ Go to the lowest floor of your home, away from glass windows or doors.
- ✓ Go to your basement and seek shelter under a stairwell and away from glass.
- ✓ If caught by the storm outside, move away from its path at a right angle.
- ✓ If walking outside, duck into a stairwell, or culvert.
- ✓ If you are outside, get inside quickly.
- ✓ If you are in a car, seek shelter immediately, even in a ditch.
- ✓ If in a building with a freestanding roof such as an auditorium or gymnasium, seek other shelter.

- ✓ If there is no time to escape, drop to the ground in the nearest ditch, ravine, or depression.
- ✓ If in a factory or warehouse, avoid walls and windows; go to a designated safe area.
- ✓ Contain pets by leash or carrier as possible.

After the Tornado

- ☐ Check for injuries and render first aid as appropriate.
- ☐ Get your heavy shoes and clothes for everyone from your emergency kits.
- ☐ Avoid driving if possible.
- ☐ If driving is necessary, proceed with caution, avoid hazards of debris and undermined roads that may collapse.
- ☐ Watch out for landslides and collapsing buildings.
- ☐ Listen to your radio or social media for information, flood warnings, and location of shelters or Red Cross stations.
- ☐ Find Red Cross disaster stations for emergency medical attention using your mobile device or social media.
- ☐ Stay away from disaster areas unless qualified to help. Leave first aid and rescue workers unhampered.
- ☐ Do not touch loose or dangling electrical wires. Report them to the power company.
- ☐ Report broken sewers and water mains to utility company.
- ☐ Stay away from river banks and streams where flooding can occur.
- ☐ Approach all animals and pets with caution.
- ☐ Keep animals contained as possible.
- ☐ Check in with your out-of-area contact person.
- ☐ Use caution when returning home or going to your emergency meeting spot.

Tornados

- ❏ Do not go into the house if it looks unstable.
- ❏ If separated from your household or family, call your out-of-area contact person.
- ❏ Check for natural gas leaks. Do not light a match.
- ❏ Check the outside of the house for damage to chimneys, wall cracks, and porch and deck stairways.

FLOODS

Floods are deluges of water that engulf and submerge normally dry land. Seasonal changes in the weather can unleash the volatility of these natural disasters. In mountain regions, early spring thaws can bring on rapid snowmelt that amplifies as flash flooding in scant minutes or hours. Dry regions can be hit hard too. In 2011, the worst flash flood in decades broke a 10-year drought and hit Queensland, Australia and 200,000 citizens with a plague of water following a disastrous 36-hour deluge of rain. Warm springs and summers are filled with the roar and relentless pounding rains of thunderstorms that glut streams, rivers, and lakes, overflowing their banks and the towns and cities built in harm's way.

Geologists continue to warn against building and dwelling on the floodplain due to its recurring and inevitable cycle of flooding. Nature's cycle has been punctuated by the sudden drama of catastrophic events. Towering tsunami waves have swept in on the heels of earthquakes and volcanic eruptions and washed away entire communities. This happened in the fall of 2010 when Indonesia's Mount Merapi erupted and triggered a devastating tsunami that ravaged the land. In 2011, another seismic catastrophe struck the east coast of Japan with a 9.0 quake that spawned a speeding ocean wave. The tsunami traveled 5,000 miles at full throttle before it swamped the island and barreled into foreign shores.

Raging windstorms have triggered flooding too, and the ocean born turbulence of hurricanes has propelled tidal waves, dumped giant cisterns of seawater on shore and sopped up vast spans of coastline. In 2005 in the United States, an explosive tropical cyclone turned into a man-made disaster and generated a massive flood. Design flaws and poor maintenance weakened the levee system and allowed it to burst under the duress of the monumental storm. The high octane winds and rains of Hurricane Katrina blasted the states of Louisiana, Mississippi, and Alabama and destroyed the old levee protecting low lying New Orleans. The floodgates of Lake Pontchartrain opened and combined with the 28-foot storm surges to cover the city and its people with 20 feet of water. One million Gulf coast residents were displaced by the disaster, and Risk Management Solutions estimates the costs will climb to $150 billion.

In 2011, history repeated itself and again spelled catastrophe in the billions for Louisiana and four neighboring states swamped by Big Muddy floodwaters. Incessant deluges of rain fattened the mighty Mississippi River to six times its normal girth and spewed thick, brown water onto shore in Missouri, Tennessee, Mississippi, and Arkansas. The inundation of water on farms and croplands was projected to rise from the normal height of 25 feet and crest up to the levee height of 47 feet. The third longest river in the world was the region's water highway and economic lifeline, and the cessation of barge traffic that had transported goods and refinery oil to market was expected to cause food and gas prices to rise.

In Arkansas where agriculture rules the economy with $16 billion in annual state revenue, *CNN Money* reported one million acres of vital crops of rice, corn, soybeans, wheat, and cotton were drowned out in the midst of high planting season. The Arkansas Farm Bureau estimated 300,000 acres would be lost, costing more than $500 million. Agricultural economists at Mississippi State University forecast $2 billion in damages to the state's grain and catfish farms alone. The losses spread to the Delta and stripped its coffers of $14 million in monthly gambling revenues when 19 casinos shut down due to flooding. Leaders of the impoverished region had lured Las Vegas-style business with low taxes and loose high stakes rules, and the gaming giants built a shimmering spread of gambling palaces in the cotton fields of Tunica, Mississippi with 1.2 million players and big profits every year. Estimates on the duration of the shutdown were approximately six to eight weeks, with worker layoffs adding 13,000 to the unemployment rolls.

In neighboring Louisiana, civil engineers took bold steps to divert the Mississippi floodwater away from densely populated cities including Baton Rouge and New Orleans. They opened the gates of the Morganza Spillway, submerging 3,000 square miles of swampland and forest of the Atchafalaya Basin down south to the Gulf of Mexico. Twenty five thousand people lost their homes and would not return. President Obama signed disaster declarations for both Mississippi and Louisiana, but high deficits prompted discussions in Congress to shift the burden of the government flood insurance program to the states. The projected recovery time for the region is slated for 2013, although the National Weather Service forecasts severe spring flooding that could impact metropolitan areas and millions of people in half of the United States.

Read about flood precautions for river, coastal, and urban areas, as well as flash flooding from the United States Search and Rescue Task Force (www.ussartf.org/flooding.htm).

Below are very specific steps to take to protect you and your household before, during, and after a flood.

Before the Flood

Inside
- ❑ Take first aid and CPR classes.
- ❑ Educate yourself on flood warning and signals.
- ❑ Contact community groups for local information and emergency contact numbers.

- Consider Mapping Your Neighborhood. See Resource Guide.
- Find out if your home is on a flood plain.
- Be aware that building on the floodplain may subject you to nature's cycle of flooding.
- Do a household inventory of your possessions.
- Contact your insurance agent for flood insurance.
- Contact the National Flood Insurance Program to see if your community qualifies for insurance.
- Get information on what to do in case of flooding at home or when traveling.
- If advised to stay in place, fill the bathtub with tap water before supply is contaminated.
- Store emergency supplies including rubber boots and gloves.
- Store sandbags, plywood, plastic sheeting, and lumber to be used shoring up your home against floodwaters.
- Store propane tanks, spray paint, gasoline cans, motor oil, and propane camp stoves on concrete floors and in outside sheds.
- Map evacuation routes and save them to your mobile device or in the cloud where household members can access them.
- Include items to take and the best safe area destinations such as motel, a friend's home, or shelter.
- Use social media to contact your household members and out-of-area contact person.
- Store printed evacuation maps and routes in your car.
- Watch news and listen to the radio for forecasts and instructions.
- Fill your car's gas tank in case of evacuation.
- Make repairs and clean up.

Floods

During the Flood

Outside
- ✓ Use your mobile device, computer, TV, or radio to get flood warning updates.
- ✓ Know that the term "flood forecast" means heavy rains may cause rivers to overflow.
- ✓ If the term "flood warning" is broadcast, be aware that flooding is now occurring or will occur soon.
- ✓ Know the term "flash flood warning" means a specified area can expect sudden floods.
- ✓ Shut off the utilities at the breaker box or unplug appliances and lights if you cannot access the electrical box.
- ✓ Prepare to follow evacuation procedures.
- ✓ Do not wait for instructions to evacuate if you see a flood approaching.
- ✓ If driving, avoid storm drains and irrigation ditches.
- ✓ Never drive around a police blockade.
- ✓ Listen to the radio, news feeds, and social media alerts for updates.
- ✓ If water is rising around your car and the car won't start, abandon your vehicle at once and get to higher ground.
- ✓ Place sandbags around your home and property before intense flooding occurs.

After the Flood
- ❑ Check for injuries and apply first aid.
- ❑ Listen to public news alerts on radio, social media outlets, and TV for emergency information and instructions.
- ❑ Wait for confirmed reports of improving conditions and safe routes home.

- ❑ Use caution in returning home.
- ❑ Avoid flood-damaged areas.
- ❑ Be cautious of pets and livestock; contain and comfort pets.

WILDFIRES

Wildfires torch the land and bring enormous devastation and damage all over the world both from natural and manmade causes. There are no national boundaries for wildfires. In 2010 in Russia, the U.N. News Service reported one million acres destroyed by wildfires (www.un.org/news). In the same year in Portugal, northeast of Lisbon, the hottest July in 80 years ignited 29 wildfires. In British Columbia, Canada and in the Yukon Territory, firefighting costs soared to $400 million per year and it is estimated that the cost of wildfire damage in the United States is roughly $3 billion per year.

Wildfires sparked by tinderbox and drought conditions are prevalent in the spring, summer, and early fall seasons. When temperatures soar and heat waves dry out vegetation, it can quickly be kindled into a fire. Leaf litter, low brush, peat, dead wood, and piles of manure from grazing animals can often break out in spontaneous combustion. Ground fires can spread from the forest floor to bridges of sapling trees and rise to a tower of flames atop forest canopies. Strong wind gusts can accelerate the flames, carrying embers and fanning the fire out through timberlands and over parched prairies. Lightning bolts hurled by electrically-charged thunderstorms are often the flint that ignites forest fires or ground fires on open land.

Lightning can also hit tall peaks, power lines, trees, transmission towers, and houses causing power outages and home fires. Other natural disasters can beget wildfires as secondary events. Cyclones conveying thunderstorms and lightning can spark fires, and volcanic eruptions with molten lava flows and hot airborne ash will set vegetation in its path on fire. Earthquakes can cause gas explosions that start fires in cities and spread to rural areas. Wildfires that leave hillsides scorched destabilize trees and vegetation causing erosion. Communities below the burned off hillsides are then at risk for mudslides, debris flow, and landslides.

Human carelessness and criminal arson have been shown to be the biggest causes of wildfires. These man-made disasters can start with the flick of a match, the toss of a lit cigarette, a spark off a gas lawnmower, the rebirth of a still smoldering campfire, a gust of wind scattering yard debris embers and shooting off fireworks near dry grass. Accidents can cause wildfires too. Trees falling and downed power lines, shorts in worn electrical lines, malfunctioning electric transformers mishaps by repair crews welding railroad tracks, accidental oil or gas leaks, and malfunctioning machinery can all be at fault.

Below are very specific steps to take to protect you and your household before, during, and after a wildfire.

Before the Wildfire

Outside
- Contact the Forestry Department for local wildfire history and guidelines.
- Identify and correct fire risks in and around your home.
- If building near forests or grasslands, use fire resistant siding and roofing.
- Use non-combustible materials: treated wood, stone, aluminum, and brick.
- Limit fuel and a pathway for a fire by planting shrubs and trees sparsely.
- Plant large trees and bushes at least 10 feet away from the house.
- Trim trees away from roofs of the house, garage, or shop.
- Remove dead or rotting tree limbs, trees, and shrubs.

Wildfires

- ❑ Trim tree branches away from power lines that could fall and ignite a fire.
- ❑ Call the electrical utility company to trim trees touching power lines.
- ❑ Keep a 30-foot firebreak of nonflammable vegetation around the house.
- ❑ Stack firewood away from the house on level ground, not downhill.
- ❑ Be aware that fires often travel uphill.
- ❑ Remove flammable mulch and moss.
- ❑ Mow lawns and cut brush regularly.
- ❑ Build decks with nonflammable materials or remove hazardous decks abutting the house.
- ❑ Install low-growth plants in landscaping.
- ❑ Water and prune landscaping well for a protective fire line near the house.
- ❑ On a hillside or forestland, clear a perimeter of 100 feet.
- ❑ Haul away yard debris regularly, before it piles up and creates a fire hazard.
- ❑ Remove and replace missing roof shingles; clean dead moss off roof.
- ❑ Replace wood shake roof with nonflammable roof materials.
- ❑ Hire a chimney sweep to remove creosote, animal nests, and debris from chimneys.
- ❑ Buy spark arrestors at a local hardware store, install in chimneys and on combustible equipment.
- ❑ Install screens on all roof vents to keep flying sparks, embers, and ash out.
- ❑ Clean gutters, roof drains, and downspouts; remove dried leaves.
- ❑ Store all flammables away from the house in sheds or outbuildings.

- Comply with local burning restrictions when disposing of yard debris.
- In rural areas, store water in tanks, wells, and cisterns to fight a fire.
- Maintain high volume pumps and hoses, and keep them close.
- In case of a power outage, have backup generator for well pumps.
- Test hoses for leaks, ensure that they reach around the perimeter of the house.
- Maintain swimming pools and ponds for water access during fire season.
- Always keep a hose with a nozzle attachment on an outside outlet.
- Stock tools to fight fire: axe, rake, chainsaw, round shovel, and bucket.
- Have a ladder tall enough to reach the top of your roof.
- Maintain two-way roads with a parking lane to give fire trucks access.
- Build roads with slopes less than 10 feet per 100 feet for easier fire truck access.
- Clear the road of flammable brush 60 feet wide along the right of way.

Inside
- Get homeowner's or renter's insurance with adequate fire coverage.
  - Inventory your possessions.
  - Update coverage after expensive purchases or remodeling.
- Attend neighborhood meetings on emergency evacuation procedures.
- Take Red Cross first aid, CPR, and fire safety classes.

Wildfires

- ❑ Call a household meeting; plan walking and driving escape routes.
- ❑ Draw a floor plan, find two exits from every room, and mark exits.
- ❑ Walk and drive evacuation and alternative routes.
- ❑ Conduct drills and practice at different times of day and night.
- ❑ Discuss livestock and pet plans, contact local shelters and motels.
- ❑ Store cage, leashes, pet carriers, pet supplies, food, water, and medications.
- ❑ Get pet licenses and vaccinations; put your name, cell phone number, and address on I.D. tags.
- ❑ See your vet to register and track pets with computer chips.
- ❑ Store portable emergency supplies, food, and water in a close by location.
- ❑ Post fire emergency numbers if different than 9-1-1.
- ❑ Install smoke detectors on every floor; test and replace batteries; and test twice a year.
- ❑ Teach children what warning sirens or home smoke alarms sound like.
- ❑ Teach children their full names, address, and phone numbers.
- ❑ Use Map Your Neighborhood for up-to-date names and phone numbers.
- ❑ Install smoke detectors in garage, workshop, and other buildings.
- ❑ Test kitchen and hallway fire extinguishers, replace as necessary.
- ❑ Get rope or chain ladders for upper stories and practice using.
- ❑ Inspect and repair doors and windows to open and close easily.

- ❑ Keep a footstool or small ladder by a non-egress window in the basement.
- ❑ Plan for special medical needs, store important prescription medications.
- ❑ If someone uses a walker, have them sleep on the ground floor.
- ❑ Install strobe light on smoke alarm to assist deaf person.

During the Wildfire

- ✓ Listen to the emergency broadcast radio for wildfire warnings/reports.
- ✓ Put heavy shoes and protective clothing on everyone.
- ✓ Use the back of your hand to test for heat before opening any door.
- ✓ Avoid opening any door that feels warm or hot.
- ✓ Close doors when exiting rooms or the house.
- ✓ Cover nose and mouth, and walk or crawl low to avoid smoke.
- ✓ Turn off gas at the meter to avoid danger of explosion.
- ✓ Take your stored supplies when evacuating.
- ✓ Use the "get out and stay out" rule. Do not return to the house in a fire.
- ✓ Travel on your preplanned route if it is confirmed to be safe.
- ✓ Use alternate walking or driving routes as necessary.
- ✓ If stranded in a car, tie a bright cloth onto the antenna.
  - If you are in a safe place, wait in your car for rescue workers.

After the Wildfire

- ❑ Administer first aid as able, or seek medical help.
- ❑ Listen to radio reports for instructions and updates of prevailing conditions.

Wildfires

- ❏ Locate disaster stations, shelters, and animal holding areas using mobile devices.
- ❏ If returning home, use caution and heed official warnings and public alerts.
- ❏ Check road conditions and use extreme caution driving or walking.
- ❏ Do not travel on roads that appear unsafe or not clear.
- ❏ Avoid wildfire damage and active fire areas.
- ❏ Know where your designated emergency staging area will be located.
- ❏ Know where an alternate disaster staging area or shelter is in case the first one is inaccessible.
- ❏ Check your home's exterior for damage and instability.
- ❏ Do not go inside if the structure appears unsafe.
- ❏ Locate anyone missing by calling your out-of-area contact.
- ❏ Access the Red Cross location service network at local disaster shelters.
- ❏ Approach animals with caution; comfort and contain them as possible.
- ❏ Check fenced areas for livestock, and repair broken fencing.

THUNDERSTORMS

Thunderstorms are the most prolific, common, and costly of storms. According to the National Weather Service (www.weather.gov), there are, at any given moment in time, 2,000 thunderstorms all over the globe with 100 lightning strikes per second and a cost of $3 billion in damages. Every day there are 45,000 thunderstorms with an annual count of 16 million thunderstorms worldwide. In the United States, where 100,000 of these thunderstorms rage every year, Florida is the most frequently assaulted state. Spring and summer are prime thunderstorm seasons, with afternoon and evening serving as the most common times of occurrence.

Generated from atmospheric temperature imbalances, these violent storms are caused by the upward transfer of heat known as convection. They can also arrive slipstreaming on the coattails of cyclones in flashing lightning, rumbling thunder, and pelting rain or hail with winds of up to 50-mph. Flash flooding is a potential aftermath of such an outburst. Because thunderstorms come to life in massive, dark tents of cumulonimbus clouds that carry electric charges, they are electrical storms wielding potentially damaging lightning bolts. The roar of thunder is the sound of rapidly expanding gases in the path of the lightning's electrical discharge.

Giant storms of 10-miles high can measure twice as wide. Separate, adjoining thunderstorms may spread out over several hundred miles to form what are known as squall lines. The storms, or cells, can continue by replacing old cells with new ones in relay fashion. Microbursts are quick, forceful surges that create hurricane-powerful, horizontal winds with speeds up to 200-mph, tackling power lines, uprooting trees, shattering windows, damaging buildings, and blowing roofs

193

off. Airplanes struck by sudden wind gusts and shifting vertical pressures have been known to crash due to their sustained structural damage.

Below are very specific steps to take to protect you and your household before, during, and after a thunderstorm.

Before the Thunderstorm

Outside
- Be aware of warning signs, seen as changes in the weather.
- Be aware that lightning is the main danger of a thunderstorm.
- Listen for thunder.
- Know if you can hear thunder, you are close enough to be struck by lightning.
- Seek shelter immediately if you are outside and you hear thunder.
- Look for darkening rain clouds and skies.
- Watch for light flashes.
- Be aware of increasing winds and lowering temperatures.
- Keep your distance from the storm.

Inside
- Attend CPR and first aid classes.
- Store supplies and water in a readily accessible place.
- Listen to news and watch weather forecasts and updates.
- Be aware of any flood warnings or watches.
- If a flood is predicted, raise furniture off floor if time permits.

During the Thunderstorm

Outside
- ✓ Take cover in a building or a car, not in a convertible.
- ✓ If in the woods, take cover under shorter trees.
- ✓ If in the water, swimming or in a boat, get to land and look for shelter.
- ✓ Listen to a portable radio or check mobile devices or Internet for news and instructions.
- ✓ Keep away from trees, metal objects, or poles.
- ✓ Squat low to the ground, tuck head in between knees. Become a small target.
- ✓ Do not lie flat on the ground.
- ✓ Get pets and livestock contained; put dogs on a leash, cats in a carrier.

Inside
- ✓ Know electricity can be conducted through phone lines and metal pipes.
- ✓ Unplug appliances.
- ✓ Check portable radio or cell phone alerts for storm news and warnings.
- ✓ Do not run water, bathe, or shower due to dangers from lightening and electrical shock.
- ✓ Turn off air conditioning to avoid damage from surges.
- ✓ Pull window shades or close blinds to protect from shattering window glass.
  - Know that forceful winds can blow objects into windows.

After the Thunderstorm

- Check for injuries and apply first aid.
- Be aware persons struck by lightning do not retain an electrical charge.
- Check on lightning victims. Check for entry and exit burns and treat accordingly.
- Administer CPR to the victim, if you are trained to render this aid.
- Listen to the radio or check your cell phone for news and instructions.
- Follow instructions on locations of emergency medical aid.
- Check on holding areas for lost pets and livestock.
- Avoid storm-damaged and flooded areas.
- Be cautious of pets and other animals; contain your own pets.
- Repair broken windows, downed fences, and fallen chimneys.
- Report downed power lines, sewer damage to utility company hotlines.
- Wait for confirmed reports on road damage and safe emergency routes before returning home.
- Wait the storm out. Use caution driving or traveling on foot.

BLIZZARDS

Winter is the most common time of year for blizzards to break out, and the cold seasons of countries around the globe vary with their regional climates. Blizzards typically appear in the northern United States east of the Rocky Mountains, especially around the Great Lakes region and in Canada. A blizzard is a tempestuous, frigid snowstorm with blustery, piercing winds of 35-mph or more and a wind-chill factor as low as -20 degrees Fahrenheit. Whiteouts, when the air is filled with so much snow that the earth and sky cannot be distinguished, have been known to blind animals and humans. Not knowing up from down can disorient livestock, drive them away from their quarters, and cause them to freeze to death.

People's lives can also be threatened by the hostile, freezing elements of a blizzard. Those traveling through mountainous areas have been stranded when their cars got stuck in snowdrifts on back roads. Hikers and skiers out for a day of recreation have run into the icy blasts and turmoil of sudden storms and succumbed to hypothermia, frost bite, and suffocation. Daytrips have ended in tragedy numerous times in the Mt. Hood region of Oregon's Cascade Range in the United States. Both the experienced and inexperienced have been overtaken by deadly blizzard conditions.

Arctic temperatures escalate the dangers of the storms in mountainous regions. Recorded temperatures diving below zero degrees with winds of up to 100-mph have imperiled all who would tread there—man and beast alike. You can view wind-chill charts at the United States Search and Rescue Task Force website (www.ussartf.org/blizzards.htm) along with detailed explanations on blizzard dangers.

Below are some preventive steps to take before, during, and after a blizzard.

Before the Blizzard

Outside

It is best to stay inside, but if you must go out, take the following precautions against the elements, frostbite, and hypothermia:

- ❑ Be aware that several lightweight layers of clothing provide more warmth than one heavy coat.
- ❑ Layer up. As an example, put on thermal underwear first, a turtleneck, a medium sweater, and then a jacket.
  - Wear a hat to prevent major heat loss from the top of your head.
- ❑ Cover your mouth so that your lungs are protected and wear gloves.
- ❑ Know the wind-chill factor.
- ❑ Be aware that wind and very cold temperatures on skin can rapidly drive down body temperatures.
- ❑ Be careful to avoid falling if walking on snow and icy sidewalks.
- ❑ Wear heavy snow or hiking boots, golf shoes, or put duct tape on the bottom of shoes.
- ❑ Sprinkle rock salt, sand, or kitty litter on slippery paths.
- ❑ In snow country, tell someone where you are going, your destination and route, and your expected arrival and return time.
- ❑ Be aware of the risks of hypothermia, frostbite, and getting stranded.
- ❑ Avoid driving the car if possible, but prepare the car for evacuation if needed.
  - Keep gas tank filled in case evacuation is ordered.
  - Keep supplies in the car's trunk, including warm blankets, coats, gloves, hats, boots, flares, and a cell phone with a crank charger.

Blizzards

- ☐ Include a shovel, sand, rope, tire chains, jumper cables, and a bright signal cloth for the car's antenna.
- ☐ Have your car winterized. Flush the radiator; add antifreeze.
  - Check the battery, electrical system, and headlights.
- ☐ Clear snow away from walking areas.
- ☐ Uncover fire hydrants, road signs, address numbers, street signs.
- ☐ Store firewood and refill the heating fuel supply as needed.

Inside

- ☐ Store emergency supplies and water in a readily accessible place.
- ☐ Take first aid and CPR classes.
- ☐ Check and apply insulation around interior pipes.
- ☐ Wrap and strap hot water heater, as shown online (www.energysavers.gov).
- ☐ Have chimney flue cleaned out annually to prevent fire.
- ☐ Shut rooms off or heat only one room to conserve heat.
- ☐ Insulate attic.
- ☐ Insulate around doors, windows, and outlets.
- ☐ Roll blankets or towels up and stuff under doors to block cold.
- ☐ Install storm windows—plastic or shutters.
- ☐ Hang blankets or drapes over windows to keep cold air out.

During the Blizzard

Outside

- ✓ Listen to a portable radio or check social media for storm warnings.

- ✓ In case of a storm watch, be aware that a storm is possible.
- ✓ In case of a storm warning, head back towards shelter.
- ✓ In case of a blizzard warning, take shelter immediately.
- ✓ If you get stuck in a car, stay with the car.
  - Tie the bright cloth onto the car's antenna for rescuers to see.
  - Keep a window cracked for air.
  - Stay warm by moving your arms and legs while sitting.
  - Start car once per hour, use heater for 10 minutes.
  - Leave dome light on while engine runs.
  - Check exhaust pipe to make sure it's not blocked by any debris or objects.
- ✓ Contain pets by leash or carrier.

Inside
- ✓ Have the warm water dripping to prevent frozen pipes.
- ✓ Monitor the storm on newsfeeds, radio, TV, Twitter, or Facebook.
- ✓ Gather stored supplies for use.
- ✓ Secure doors and windows.
- ✓ Know the signs of frostbite and hypothermia.
- ✓ Prepare to give first aid to those returning from outdoors.
- ✓ Stay inside if it is safe to do so.

After the Blizzard
- ❑ Check for injuries and apply first aid.
- ❑ Approach pets with caution; comfort and aid them.
- ❑ Repair any broken water pipes.
- ❑ Check chimney for structural damage and make repairs.
- ❑ Repair or seal and board up any broken windows.

Blizzards

- ❏ Call utility company to report downed power lines.
- ❏ Check news alerts for emergency updates or to get medical aid.
- ❏ Avoid storm damaged areas.
- ❏ Check yard for damaged fencing or downed power lines before returning pets to the yard.
- ❏ Check for locations of holding areas for lost pets or livestock through sites such as Facebook, The Humane Society, and Red Cross.
- ❏ Contain pets and livestock for at least one to two days after an event.

CYCLONES

Cyclones are related to other swashbuckling rotary storms like hurricanes that arise from warm ocean waters, but these tropical cyclones blast in from the cold. The storms are born high over frozen Siberia with intensifying low-pressure systems that can ascend to 30,000 feet. The lumbering giants can grow to a width of 1,000 miles in diameter. Their wildly revolving winds blow at between 20 to 50-mph around a calm center called the eye of the storm. Within their one week lifespans, cyclones can deliver prolonged blizzards and bitter stints of snow and icy rain to a wide geographic breadth.

In North America, the swirling storms break out east of the Rockies and in the central and northeastern regions of the United States. In the southern hemisphere, they spawn destructive vortexes over the Pacific Ocean to the east and south of Japan. Cyclones travel long routes all the way north from their points of origin, cruising along on a northeast track from there and they fly aloft, dumping frigid loads of punishing winter weather like meteorological bombardiers. Cyclones that begin in the Gulf of Mexico mobilize along the eastern coast and onto the North Atlantic Ocean, while those beginning in Spain strike the Mediterranean and Europe, and they also form in the Indian Ocean around Australia. Here, the direction of the winds' rotation changes and they blow in a counterclockwise direction, circulating around the placid center. Although cyclones do not always carry precipitation, they do bring an arsenal of thunderstorms and showers to warm climates. For a definition of cyclones, hurricanes, and typhoons, go online to the National Weather Service website (http://www.srh.noaa.gov/srh/jetstream/tropics/tc.htm).

Below are steps for dealing with a cyclone before, during, and after it occurs.

Before the Cyclone

Outside

- ❑ Watch the weather; look for darkening skies, rising wind, rain torrents.
- ❑ Watch for blizzard conditions, ice and snow.
- ❑ Get inside or seek other shelter immediately.
- ❑ If in a car, pull over and wait the storm out. Stay warm.
- ❑ If at the beach, watch for waves coming inland. Stay alert for thunderstorms in warm climates.
- ❑ Leave low-lying areas due to the danger of floods and high tides.
- ❑ If swimming or in a boat, get to shore and seek shelter. Secure the boat or evacuate to a predetermined safe area.
- ❑ Secure or take inside: garbage cans, children's toys, lawn furniture, gardening tools, barbecues, or any object the wind could hurl.
- ❑ Fill your car's gas tank in case of evacuation.
- ❑ Check news sources by TV, radio, cell phone, or Internet for instructions.
- ❑ Board up windows, close shutters, tape glass.
- ❑ Be aware that wind pressure can shatter large windows and flying debris can break smaller panes of glass.
- ❑ Contain pets and livestock in a safe area.

Inside

- ❑ Get insurance and inventory your possessions.
- ❑ Secure this information where you can retrieve it in case you file a claim.
- ❑ Take first aid and CPR classes; attend community meetings.
- ❑ Listen for storm advisories and warnings on TV, radio, Internet.

Cyclones

- ❑ Check your camping equipment, emergency cooking equipment, and water and food supply.
- ❑ Have cold weather gear, hats, gloves, and boots on hand.
- ❑ Secure your home. Move to the side of the house away from the wind.
- ❑ Check flashlights, gather portable radio, fresh batteries, and cell phone hand crank chargers.
- ❑ Store water before the supply can be contaminated.
- ❑ Fill clean jugs, pans, and even the bathtub with water.
- ❑ If you are in a mobile home, or in an RV park, leave as soon as you hear the storm warning. Go to a designated shelter.
- ❑ Evacuate according to official instructions and follow safe routes.

During the Cyclone

- ✓ If your home is stable and sturdy, stay in and wait out the storm.
- ✓ Beware of the eye, the calm center of the storm, as it passes overhead.
  - Be aware that the calm may last from two minutes to half an hour.
- ✓ If you have a basement or storm cellar, wait out the storm there.
- ✓ If you do not have a basement, go to the lowest floor of your home, away from glass windows or doors.
- ✓ Contain pets by leash or carrier.

After the Cyclone

- ❑ Check for injuries, treat yourself first.
- ❑ Avoid driving if possible.
  - If driving is necessary, drive with caution. Avoid

hazards, debris, and roads that could be undermined and collapse.
- ❑ Check public alerts for information such as flood warnings, location of shelters, and Red Cross stations.
- ❑ Know locations of neighborhood or community emergency staging areas, alternatives.
- ❑ Stay away from disaster scenes unless qualified to help. First aid and rescue workers will function best unhampered.
- ❑ Use caution when returning home and approaching animals.
- ❑ Do not touch loose or dangling electrical wires.
- ❑ Report shorting wires and power outages to the power company.
- ❑ Be aware that cyclones moving inland may bring severe flooding.
- ❑ Stay away from river banks and streams where flooding and landslides can occur.

TYPHOONS

Typhoons are spawned in the warm ocean close to the heart of the Equator. These tropical cyclones are hurricane-like storms that arise in the western Pacific as tropical depressions, and they can evolve into more powerful storms in the oceans between the latitudes of 5 and 20 degrees North and South. The stormy existence of typhoons is guided by the trade winds that navigate their paths. Typhoons develop and grow where the temperature of the sea measures 80 degrees Fahrenheit or more, most commonly in the warmer weather of summer and fall. Their average lifespan is roughly ten days, and their whirling winds and rains can broadcast wild destruction.

In October 2010, super typhoon Megi bombarded the Philippines and northeast Luzon Island with high velocity uproar. The category-five storm spread catastrophic wreakage and downed vital power and communication lines. Seven thousand people were evacuated and 19 were killed. *Euro News* reported that the tropical cyclone picked up more momentum as it headed for the South China Sea and on to Hong Kong. Tracking weather changes is done by satellites, and the National Oceanic and Atmospheric Administration (www.noaa.gov) provides climate services data and satellite information for real time, up-to-date weather news, especially regarding typhoons.

Below are steps for protecting you and your household before, during, and after a typhoon.

Before the Typhoon

Outside
- ❑ Watch the weather; look for darkening skies, rising wind, rain torrents.

- ❏ If at the beach, watch for waves coming inland, stay alert.
- ❏ Leave low-lying areas due to danger from high tides and flooding.
- ❏ If swimming or in a boat, get to shore. Secure the boat in a pre-designated safe area and seek shelter.
- ❏ Secure or take inside: garbage cans, children's toys, lawn furniture, gardening tools, barbecues, or any object the wind could hurl.
- ❏ Fill your car's gas tank.
- ❏ Check for public alerts by radio or check social media for news and updates.
- ❏ Board up windows, close shutters, tape glass.
- ❏ Be aware that wind pressure can shatter large windows and flying debris can break smaller panes of glass.
- ❏ Contain pets and livestock.

Inside
- ❏ Get insurance and inventory your possessions.
  - Secure this information where you can retrieve it in case you file a claim.
- ❏ Attend community meetings; take first aid and CPR classes.
- ❏ Listen for storm advisories and warnings on TV, radio, and Internet.
- ❏ Check your food, water, camping equipment, and emergency supplies.
- ❏ Secure your home. Move to the side of the house away from the wind.
- ❏ Check flashlights and portable radio, cell phones, and crank chargers.
- ❏ Store water before the supply can be contaminated. Use

soda bottles, clean jugs, pans, and even the bathtub as containers.
- ❑ If you are in a mobile home, leave the premises as soon as you hear the storm warning. Go to a designated shelter.
- ❑ Evacuate according to instructions.

During the Typhoon

- ✓ If your home is secure, stay in and wait out the storm.
- ✓ If you have a basement or storm cellar, wait out the storm there.
- ✓ If you do not have a basement, go to the lowest floor of your home. Stay away from glass windows or doors.
- ✓ Beware of the eye, the calm center of the storm, as it passes overhead.
  - Be aware that the calm can last from two minutes to half an hour.
- ✓ Contain pets by leash or carrier.

After the Typhoon

- ❑ Check for injuries and render first aid.
- ❑ Avoid driving if possible. If driving is necessary, drive with caution.
- ❑ Avoid hazards, debris, and undermined roads that may collapse.
- ❑ Be aware that landslides are also possible.
- ❑ Be aware that typhoons moving inland can bring severe flooding and stay clear of water ways.
- ❑ Check social media, TV, or radio for information and flood warnings.
- ❑ Check the location of shelters and Red Cross Disaster Stations.

- ❏ Go to Red Cross disaster stations for emergency medical attention.
- ❏ Stay away from disaster areas unless qualified to help. Let first aid and rescue workers work unhampered.
- ❏ Use caution when returning home.
- ❏ Do not enter your house if it appears damaged or unsafe.
- ❏ Do not touch loose or dangling electrical wires.
- ❏ Report shorted wires to the power company.
- ❏ Stay away from river banks and streams where flooding can occur.
- ❏ Keep animals contained long enough to calm them, even a few days.
- ❏ Make repairs and clean up.

Man-Made Disasters

Like natural disasters, man-made disasters break out everywhere in the world, suddenly propelling communities, countries, or large geographic regions into states of emergency. Industrial-level accidents occur randomly, outside the normal course of events, and they can impact large populations. Pesticide plant explosions and a multitude of other toxic chemical releases from factories and refineries have delivered both immediate and long-term harm. Enormous destruction and chaos can be caused by human beings making mistakes in judgment. The mix of human error and equipment failure has culminated in nuclear power plant meltdowns and radioactive releases with devastating effects.

The issue of poor worker training has been raised in response to mine waste leaks that polluted water supplies for millions and power blackouts that plunged major cities into darkness and deadlock. Mismanagement of inclement weather conditions has left travelers, skiers, and outdoor enthusiasts stranded and, at worst, with their lives at risk. Negligence has proved deadly when weak dams and levees burst under the duress of powerful storms, flooding the cities and inhabitants below.

In addition, sudden accidents can happen anywhere hazardous materials are being stored or transported. The roadways, rivers, oceans, and railways that carry hazardous materials to their destinations are vulnerable to a long list of unforeseen accidents. Virtually anywhere tankers, freighters, buses, and trains travel with their cargo a man-made disaster can happen, bringing long-term damage and pollution to the surrounding terrain, ecosystems, and nearby communities. Runaway freight trains have derailed and spilled their toxic cargo on sleeping towns. Offshore drilling rigs have exploded, killing crew members, polluting the environment, and stifling the economy. Sea born oil tankers have crashed into ice bergs and other tankers and fouled water and land with massive raw petroleum slicks.

Dams bursting, crashing tankers and oil spills, toxic chemical spills and explosions, power blackouts, and nuclear radiation leaks are all examples of man-made disasters that have occurred and will continue to have an impact on people and the planet. From the beginning of the industrial age, hazardous materials and modern technology have improved civilization everywhere. In a chemical and electrically dependent world the technological benefits of these resources do outweigh the harms but caution is in order. This section of the book will help you to become informed, prepare for, and learn the tactics necessary to survive any man-made disasters you may encounter.

BOMBINGS AND EXPLOSIONS

Explosions are dynamic, mega-force releases of energy that discharge in thunderous blasts. They have been used in both military and in civilian applications in war and peace, and they have a long history. Alchemists in search of an elixir of immortality had experimented with various recipes from fuels and ores. In ancient China around 850 A.D., the gunpowder concoction was discovered. The explosive mixture of sulfur, charcoal, and saltpeter was used in bombs fired from military catapults during the Tang Dynasty. Over time, during the Song and Yuan Dynasties, gunpowder was commonly detonated in cannons, rockets, and missiles used in wars. In the 12th and 13th centuries, the lethal weaponry spread to Arab countries, then to Europe and onto battlefields all over the world.

Experimentation by chemists continued. In Turin, Italy Ascano Sobrero produced an exothermic reaction by adding both nitric acid and sulphuric acid to gycero, inventing Nitroglycerin. A crystalline substance called TNT was invented in Germany by Joseph Wilbard in 1865 and was then used in mining and quarrying and later as military munitions during World War I. In the mid 1800's, the Swedish chemist Alfred Nobel solved the instability problem of Nitroglycerin by adding an absorbent powder called kieselguhr to the liquid to form a paste which could be rolled into rods and placed in drilling holes. He called this substance Dynamite and mass-produced it in his remote factory in Glasgow, Scotland. Nobel also invented the blasting cap and made his fortune in sales to the civil engineering and mining industries. Later, dynamite was prolifically used in weapons of war. At the end of his life, the man known as the father of explosives founded the Nobel Peace Prize, making it his legacy.

Over several centuries, scientific advances have harnessed

the power of these substances and utilized them in a multitude of ways. The principles of managed explosions and controlled combustion of petroleum products like gasoline and vaporous mixtures produced the internal combustion engine and the Diesel engine—a boon for the development of the automobile, the bus, the tractor, the train, and the airplane. Beyond mass transit and daily commerce, the technology has also benefited mining, agriculture, infrastructure, construction, and the energy industries. Mining operations have extracted not only precious ores but also coal, gas, and oil for energy usage. Explosives opened up quarries and allowed construction interests access to the raw building materials for homes, factories, and cities. Farmlands cleared by explosive blasting yielded food and grain, and raised livestock.

Central to production of crops and herds was access to water by irrigation systems of drainage ditches, canals, and aqueducts dug out from the land by blasting. Dams have also been built as a result of excavation by explosives. Construction of the transportation network of roads, highways, tunnels, bridges, and railroads has all been made possible by blasting through the use of dynamite and other chemicals. This infrastructure has not only transported harvests from farms to market, it has opened up the world of economic commerce.

Other uses of explosives have included disaster relief from both natural and man-made causes. In 1985, explosives were used in the rescue and clean-up following the Mexico City earthquake that killed 5,000 people. In 1992 after the Persian Gulf War, explosive charges helped extinguish the 700 oil well fires set by Iraq leader Saddam Hussein's troops in Kuwait. Explosives were also a big part of the rescue effort of the Chilean miners trapped for more than three months underground in 2010.

Bombings and Explosions

However, explosives are best known for their use by the military as weapons in wartime. Fighter planes launch air strikes against enemy targets, dropping bombs loaded with incendiary chemicals that blow up on impact. The fireball blasts dig deep craters, gouge the countryside, decimate cities, and raise hefty death tolls. Public exposure to bombs and explosions has been largely media fueled in movies, on TV, and online.

Terrorist warfare against unarmed civilians has been waged on many continents, devastating nations and their citizens. In 1983, the United States Marine barracks in Beirut, Lebanon were pulverized by a six-ton truck bomb; 241 soldiers were killed as they slept in their bunks. A simultaneous attack killed 58 French troops. In 1995 in the United States, a Ryder truck bomb blew up the Murrah Federal Building and a daycare center in Oklahoma City with a death toll of 168 men, women, and children.

Tragic school shootings also rocked the United States in the late 1990s. In 1998, a suspended senior at Thurston High School in Springfield, Oregon shot and killed both his parents with his father's semi-automatic rifle. The next day he opened fire on his fellow students in the school cafeteria killing two and wounding 25. Columbine High School in Littleton, Colorado was the scene of bloody violence in 1999 when two students killed 11 others and shot themselves dead on campus. In 2007, on the eight-year anniversary of the Columbine assault, a lone gunman carried out the most devastating campus rampage in American history. The alienated student turned shooter struck on the campus of the Virginia Polytechnic Institute, killing 33 students.

In 2001, the United States suffered the most dramatic and outrageous terrorist attack ever, when Saudi terrorists hijacked four commercial jets, flying two into the World ade Center's twin towers and crashing the third into the Pentagon, detonating the planes as bombs. The fourth jet crashed and burned in a field in Pennsylvania after passengers overtook their captors and derailed their plan to target the Pentagon. A total of nearly 3,000 lives were taken. President George W. Bush declared a war on terrorism and vowed to bring mastermind Osama bin Laden to justice. A decade later, on May 2, 2011, the manhunt ended when United States Joint Special Operations Command forces shot and killed the al-Qaeda leader in his compound inside Abbottabad, Pakistan. President Barak Obama made the announcement on the national news and called it a significant victory.

Across the Atlantic, the city of London has endured a long and violent campaign of IRA bombings since 1993. Truck bombings at the hands of Chechen rebels in Moscow have repeatedly hit the Russian government. In the face of all the bloody battles, explosives are largely regarded as deadly and destructive forces. Due to this increase in violence, the private sector has sprung into action with services that alert users to a terrorist attack via cell phone (www.nationalterroralert.com).

Below are several ways to protect yourself and your loved ones in the event of a bombing or explosion.

Before a Bombing or Explosion

Inside
- ❏ Learn first aid at the Red Cross, fire station, local community center, or college.
- ❏ If you are on a college campus, know contact methods by phone and computer for Campus Security.
- ❏ If you live or work in a high-rise building, find fire extinguishers on every floor.

Bombings and Explosions

- ❏ Learn to use an ABC extinguisher and check pressure, corrosion, and expiration date.
- ❏ Repair or replace defective fire extinguishers annually.
- ❏ Locate fire exits and review evacuation procedures where you work.
- ❏ Review workplace emergency plans.
- ❏ Find out who will be the emergency commander, and the chain of command.
- ❏ Determine which elevators are locked down, if any, where you live or work.
- ❏ Be aware exiting a building after an explosion will be by stairway.
- ❏ Store rope ladders on-site to use when fire exits or stairways are blocked.
- ❏ Determine floor and location of the office emergency kit.
- ❏ Use emergency signals and code words to alert coworkers to call 9-1-1 in case of a bomb threat or explosion.
- ❏ Put together an office emergency kit with a radio, flashlight, and signal whistle.
- ❏ Tape extra batteries to the radio and flashlight.
- ❏ Create a school emergency kit.
- ❏ Put a small emergency kit in your car.
- ❏ Keep a hard hat, heavy work gloves, and sturdy shoes in the kit.
- ❏ Include fluorescent tape to cordon off hazardous areas.
- ❏ Use duct tape to seal broken windows.
- ❏ Include a first aid kit and manual, extra prescription medications, and eyeglasses.
- ❏ Keep evacuation route map in kit.
- ❏ Pick a safe place to duck into in case of falling debris from above.

- ❏ Pick a place to take shelter in, under a sturdy desk or table, or in a closet.
- ❏ Be aware that smoke and gas from an explosion rises and collects on ceilings.
- ❏ In case of fire and smoke, know how to crawl low on the floor to avoid toxic gases.

During a Bombing or Explosion

- ✓ In a bomb threat or warning, stay away from any suspicious packages.
- ✓ Never touch or move a bomb or other explosive device.
- ✓ Keep other people away from the dangerous area, cordon off with tape.
- ✓ Notify work managers or school authorities of suspicious device(s) and location.
  - Clear the area around the suspicious package, letter or object.
- ✓ If anyone's safety is threatened by an explosion, exit immediately.
- ✓ If advised to evacuate the area, assist those with disabilities, follow instructions.
- ✓ Get quickly to designated assembly area 300 feet or more from the explosive.
- ✓ If you answer the phone at work and it is a bomb threat, stay calm.
  - Signal coworkers to call 9-1-1, notify management and call security.
  - Keep the caller on the line as long as possible.
  - Write down date and time of the call.
  - Write down exactly what is said.
  - Get as much information as possible.
  - Try to determine caller's gender and age.

Bombings and Explosions

- Listen for clues as to caller's location and report details to police.
- Listen for caller's voice characteristics, background music, and noise.
- Listen for church bells, foghorns, train whistles, machinery sounds, etc.

✓ In case of an explosion in the building, stay calm and duck under a desk or table.
✓ If you are calling 9-1-1, state, "This is an emergency" and give your name and location.
  - Give the operator a brief description of what is happening.
  - Do not hang up unless your safety is threatened.
✓ If on a college campus or at a school, also call campus security.
✓ If you are at home and there is an explosion nearby, take cover.
  - Protect yourself from flying glass and debris by ducking under a table or desk.
✓ Listen to the radio and public alert systems for news bulletins and instructions.
✓ In case a fire breaks out, crawl low on the floor under smoke or toxic fumes.
✓ Cover your mouth with a wet cloth to limit smoke inhalation.
✓ If you come to a closed door, test the temperature with the back of your hand.
✓ Do not open a hot door; find another way out.
✓ If the door is not hot, open it slowly while bracing yourself against it.
✓ Stay clear of breaking windows and glass or hazards falling from above.

- ✓ Prepare to evacuate the building or home as directed by authorities.

After a Bombing or Explosion

- ❑ Evacuate the building or home as directed by authorities, follow instructions.
- ❑ Steer clear of outward shattering windows from high-rise buildings.
- ❑ Leave the sidewalks clear for emergency responders and for your safety.
- ❑ Proceed to an area a safe distance away.
- ❑ Do not go back into the building, school, or home until directed by authorities.
- ❑ If trapped in debris, use your flashlight or whistle as a signal for help.
  - Tap on a wall or pipe to signal your location.
  - Stay in the same spot and keep as still as possible.
  - Avoid shouting and breathing in toxic dust and smoke.
- ❑ Use your handkerchief, shirt, or coat to cover your nose and mouth to help avoid inhaling fumes.
- ❑ Wet a cloth for washing wounds or to cover your mouth.
- ❑ Administer first aid to yourself first; help others as possible.
- ❑ Notify your out-of-area contact person to update him or her on your situation.

NUCLEAR OCCURRENCES

Radioactive energy is in the air and all around, its atoms moving in particles, rays, and waves—invisible and undetectable. Uranium deposits in the soil, the cosmic rays of the sun, bodies of water, and the atmosphere all give off radioactive energy. People and animals carry trace amounts of it in their bodies. Modern science has harnessed this viable energy in the form of nuclear power, enhancing the daily lives of ordinary people.

Beyond the benefits of nuclear energy usage in heating and electrical plants, kitchen microwave ovens, televisions, dental X-rays, and medical tests, the specter of its risks have also emerged. The threat of a nuclear meltdown became all too real when three fueling units at the Fukushima Dai-Ichi nuclear power plant lost power and cooling after the devastating magnitude 9.0 earthquake struck Japan on March 11, 2011. Without power pumping water to cool the fuel rods at the heart of the four reactors, deadly radiation escaped in a release that rivaled the monumental nuclear disaster that befell Chernobyl, Ukraine in 1986. It was the worst calamity to endanger Japan since WWII.

Nuclear weapons of war made history in 1945 when the United States dropped two atomic bombs on the Japanese, ending the costly war. Headline photographs and movie reels of the backlit mushroom cloud streamed their way into human consciousness. The infamous airbrushed blimp hovering in the sky over Hiroshima and Nagasaki became part of an international photo album. Documentaries, textbooks, magazines, and poster art disseminated the image into posterity as well.

In the sober aftermath of war, a healthy fear of a nuclear bomb attack and obliteration influenced nations and curtailed WWIII. The strategic threat of weapons of mass destruction loomed large in the Cold War period and prevailed long after. In 2003, the United States and its allies launched a military campaign against Iraq based on intelligence reports of weapons of mass destruction. Even at the time of this writing, the Middle East conflict continues unresolved in Afghanistan.

Following the drama of war, nuclear science has developed its most useful applications in peacetime. Radioactive energy heats and lights homes, offices, and public buildings and provides state-of-the-art medical treatment. When managed properly, nuclear power plants can be enormously beneficial, and these utility companies operate successfully all over the world. Technical measures and strict industry regulations have been put in place to minimize risks of accidental releases of radiation.

Human error, design deficiencies, safety issues, loss of coolant, and equipment failure are the reported causes for nuclear accidents and radiation threats. Because of this, reasonable concerns about potential nuclear power plant leaks, reactor meltdowns, and other accidental releases of harmful or lethal doses of radiation should exist—both within the public and by regulators. Nuclear reactor meltdowns come at a high dollar, environmental and human cost. The worst commercial nuclear plant release in the United States took place in 1979. Located in Pennsylvania, Three Mile Island had a partial reactor meltdown due to a loss of coolant (www.threemileisland.org). No one was killed or injured, and exposure to the general population of two million was estimated to be less than a chest X-ray. The economic cost of the disaster was a significant $2.4 million. Investigators found an alarming trio of causes of the accident: design deficiencies, worker error, and component failures. These findings spurred permanent and sweeping changes in the nuclear industry and to the Nuclear Regulatory Commission (NRC).

In 1986, the Chernobyl nuclear reactor meltdown in Ukraine made history as the most momentous man-made disaster ever recorded. The death toll was projected at 4,000 by the International Atomic Energy Agency and the cost was $6.7 million. On top of that, 350,000 people were forcibly removed from the contaminated area, and a 30-mile radius was cleared around the closed plant. Radioactivity was released all over the Soviet Union and carried by winds all over Europe (www.world-nuclear.org). In 2009, three respected Russian nuclear scientists released a book, *Chernobyl: Consequences of the Catastrophe for People and the Environment,* and calculated 985,000 deaths based on the health and radiological data they studied. Other controversy surfaced when, 25 years after the radioactive disaster, it was announced that the defunct nuclear plant would open to tour groups visiting Russia in 2011.

The nation of Japan has endured repeated nuclear reactor incidents. In 2004 in Fukui, Japan, steam explosions rocked the Mihama Nuclear Power Plant and cost five people their lives, injuring dozens with a price tag of $9 million. Later in Japan, in 2007, a nuclear power plant unwittingly built on top of an active seismic fault was struck by a magnitude 6.8 earthquake. Pipes burst, radiation was released, and fires broke out.

The medical uses of nuclear energy are by and large a great boon to civilization, although some serious radiotherapy accidents have been reported. The causes have ranged from transportation mishaps to equipment failure and safety problems and human error. Sources of radiation have been misplaced, lost, stolen, sold for scrap, or abandoned. In

Mexico City, four patients died due to accidental radiation overdoses in 1984. In San Jose, Costa Rica 13 fatalities and 114 radiation injuries to hospital patients were suffered in 1996. In 1999 in Tokaimura, Japan an irradiation accident critically exposed 27 workers, with acute health effects to 119 people that resulted in two fatalities.

In addition, the medical uses of nuclear energy can have damaging effects even after leaving the medical system. According to the International Atomic Energy Agency, the scrap metal industry is one of the biggest harbors of radiation accidents. In 1987, the worst radiation disaster in the Western Hemisphere injured 244 and killed four people in Goiania, Brazil. The contamination came from Cesium-137 in a cancer therapy machine sold as scrap. In Mayapuri, India in 2010, a cobalt 60 radiation source sold to a scrap metal dealer at auction caused one death and a number of hospitalizations for radiation sickness.

On an everyday basis, humans are exposed to trace amounts of radioactive energy, but in a nuclear disaster, human exposure to radiation is a threat and lethal doses are possible. Such an event is highly survivable if the correct actions are taken to minimize exposure. According to the director of preparedness at the National Security Council, the safest way to avoid serious nuclear contamination is to take shelter inside within the first 60 minutes of nuclear exposure. The aim is to limit external exposure by shielding against high levels of radioactivity. Not breathing in contaminated air and not ingesting exposed food and water will help lessen internal exposure. Limiting either type of exposure will help maximize survival and minimize injury.

Health and mortality can be threatened in lesser or greater degrees depending on the amount and type of radiation absorbed by the body and the length of time of the exposure.

For example, workers in a nuclear power plant where a reactor meltdown happens would have a higher degree of exposure to a critical dose of radiation than those living 30 miles away from the site of the accident. It is important to know that radiation cannot be recognized by sight, smell, or taste. It is critical to observe your surroundings, carefully analyzing the situation. If you see someone on the ground choking or having a seizure, a heart attack may be the most likely cause of the symptoms. If you see a number of individuals on the ground coughing or vomiting, they may be reacting to a radioactive substance. Evaluate the scene and alert authorities as quickly as possible. Do not try to aid victims of a nuclear accident until authorities indicate it is safe, and the source has been identified and isolated.

Below are action steps you can take to protect yourself in the event of a nuclear occurrence.

Before a Nuclear Occurrence

Inside
- Attend neighborhood, community, and public meetings.
- Be aware that taking cover inside is better than evacuation in most cases.
- Limit exposure to any sources of radiation.
- Find nuclear safety and emergency information in utility bills and from FEMA.
- Check community calendars for meetings and workshops on nuclear emergencies.
- Review nearby nuclear power plant emergency plans.
- Know that 10 to 50 miles around a nuclear facility is a high-risk zone.
- Get information on health risks to children, pregnant women, and the elderly.

- ❑ Find out what the warning system is for a nuclear accident.
- ❑ Teach the warning system to household members, children.
- ❑ Register handicapped and disabled individuals with local emergency services.
- ❑ Prepare ahead to receive emergency alerts and instruction online and on cell phones.
- ❑ Pre-set car radio and cell phones to the Emergency Alerts Station.
- ❑ Know locations of local hospitals and clinics.
- ❑ Find out about workplace emergency plan(s) and evacuation routes.
- ❑ Check school's emergency plans and supplies on hand.
- ❑ Review school's plan on relocating students to a designated safe area.
- ❑ Check on apartment community emergency plan, supply kit.
- ❑ Check on retirement home emergency plans, procedures.
- ❑ Find temporary shelter for pets through veterinarian links or social media sites.
- ❑ In case evacuation is mandated, check for temporary lodging a safe distance away, up to 75 miles if near the radiation release.
- ❑ Take first aid classes and learn CPR.
- ❑ Learn about health risks and management.
- ❑ Learn about radioactivity safety precautions.
- ❑ Put together emergency kits for home, school, office, and vehicles.
- ❑ Include a change of clothing in car or at work in case you are contaminated by radiation.

- ☐ Synchronize your household and family plan using your phone and Internet.
- ☐ In first aid kit have essential prescription medications, spare eyeglasses.
- ☐ Keep cash and coins in emergency kits.
- ☐ Store canned food, water, and supplies.
- ☐ Have black plastic bags available to dispose of contaminated clothes.
- ☐ Have plastic sheets and duct tape on hand for sealing windows, vents.
- ☐ Ensure you have an out-of-area contact person to relay messages and important medical, insurance, and financial information.
- ☐ Ask your doctor if you are allergic to potassium iodine which is often given to people with radiation exposure.
- ☐ Locate a safe place to take cover—such as a basement or interior room.

During a Nuclear Occurrence

- ✓ Know if you see birds falling from the sky, it could indicate that radiation is present.
- ✓ Be aware that radiation cannot be detected by sight, smell, or touch.
- ✓ Limit the amount of time spent near the source of radiation, shelter inside.
- ✓ Do not call 9-1-1 unless it is a life or death emergency.
- ✓ Use public alerts on your cell phone or computer to track emergency announcements.
- ✓ Be aware that radioactive material loses strength quickly over time.
- ✓ If you are driving in your car, close all windows tightly, turn off vents.

Surviving Natural Disasters and Man-Made Disasters

- ✓ Shut-off AC or car heater.
- ✓ Tune in to your radio and phones for emergency information.
- ✓ If you are walking outside, get away from the accident or explosion.
  - Stay uphill, upwind, and upstream from the disaster site.
- ✓ Do not try to assist victims until authorities announce that it is safe.
- ✓ Protect yourself by taking shelter in a stable building.
- ✓ Get behind concrete and glass to shield from harmful radiation.
- ✓ Find a water source, wash off, remove, and dispose of contaminated clothes.
- ✓ If you are outside and near your home, get inside the house and stay there.
- ✓ Remove all clothing and shoes, and double seal in plastic bags.
  - Place clothing bags in garage or outside to minimize your exposure.
  - Shower off thoroughly and put on unexposed clothing.
- ✓ Close off unused rooms in your home.
  - Fill bathtub, sinks, and clean containers with extra water; turn off intake valve.
- ✓ Keep pets inside if possible.
- ✓ Close fireplace and wood stove dampers.
- ✓ Shut-off ventilation systems, heating, and cooling.
- ✓ Tightly close and secure windows, shut vents, turn off fans.
- ✓ Seal windows, vents, air ducts with tape and plastic sheeting.
- ✓ If you have a basement area or cellar, take cover there.

- ✓ Monitor the Emergency Broadcast System for updates and instructions.
- ✓ Remain inside until the all clear is given by authorities.

After a Nuclear Occurrence

- ☐ If told by authorities to stay inside at home or work, follow directions.
- ☐ Evacuate and follow directions from authorities.
- ☐ Be aware that radiation cannot be detected by sight, smell, or touch.
- ☐ Know that risk of radioactive harm is greater with closer contact and longer exposure.
- ☐ Consult your doctor on taking potassium iodide to protect your thyroid in radiation release.
  - Know that potassium iodide does not work for exposure to a dirty bomb.
  - Consult authorities for recommendations on taking potassium iodide.
- ☐ Avoid eating exposed fruits and vegetables that may be contaminated.
  - Do not eat any crops not yet harvested.
  - Wash and peel any fruits or vegetables stored inside.
- ☐ Bring pets inside if possible.
- ☐ Avoid stirring up or breathing in dust, as it may be contaminated.
- ☐ Provide as much shelter for livestock as possible, especially those producing milk.
- ☐ Give all animals previously stored feed and water.
- ☐ Store previously harvested garden crops inside.
- ☐ Use your pre-assembled emergency kits and communication devices.
- ☐ Call or text out-of-area contact person to report your situation, check on others.

TOXIC CHEMICAL RELEASES

An estimated 40,000 chemicals benefit commercial industries ranging from agriculture and energy to medicine and research. Military applications in explosives and chemical agents also serve an important purpose, but they are often overshadowed by the thousands of chemicals used in manufacturing plants and factories to produce a variety of consumer goods. These chemical agents are common in households everywhere, and they have many practical applications.

Broad, everyday uses can be ascribed to organic, petroleum-based chemicals like oil and gasoline, plastics, dyes, paints, and polyester. Inorganic cyanide, acids such as chlorine, metals, and caustic substances are frequently utilized too. That can of gasoline in the garage fuels the power mower, insecticides in the tool shed help control garden pests, and glass cleaners and bleaches disinfect the kitchen and bathroom. The drycleaner down the block removes stains from polyester clothing with solvents. Highway service stations sell gas and oil to run cars, trucks, and RVs. Automotive stores sell the rubber tires that keep motor vehicles on the asphalt road. Pool and spa outlets specialize in the sale of chlorine to kill bacteria in public and private swimming pools. In fact, the chemical is so versatile that it is also used to purify drinking water, sanitize sewage and industrial waste, and bleach paper and cloth.

These chemicals and petroleum products routinely provide enormous benefits to the modern world, but these hazardous substances are vulnerable to accidents wherever they are being mined, stored, processed, or transported. Quarries and mines, oil drilling sites, plants, factories, trains, semi-trucks, and tankers are all possible origins of hazardous releases. The oceans and rivers, oil and gas pipelines, highways and railways are also at risk for sudden toxic spills that morph into disasters. Death to human and wildlife populations, destruction of property and communities, and devastating pollution of the land, waterways, and eco systems are all possibilities in the event of a toxic chemical spill.

In 1984, one of the worst industrial accidents on record took thousands of lives in Bhopal, India (www.bhopal.com). Human error and mechanical failure led to the release of methyl isocyanate into the atmosphere. The deadly cloud of poison gas set off from the Union Carbide pesticide plant; rolling out in the early morning hours over the sleeping population. Two thousand men, women, and children died instantly, and 8,000 more fatalities followed.

In the United States just one year later, another Union Carbide plant in West Virginia accidentally released the same chemical. This second occurrence was a grim reminder that stringent improvements in mechanical, safety, and training systems were still needed. To address these inadequacies and help prevent recurrences of chemical disasters, the government stepped in. Amendments to the United States Clean Air Act in 1990 mandated worst-case scenario strategies in chemical companies' emergency plans. Other reforms soon followed (www.epa.gov/air).

On the heels of catastrophic chemical releases and hazardous spills, improvements in the industry are ongoing. Better plant design and safety controls are in progress. Innovations in green chemistry are being pursued by scientists and chemists who aim to reduce health and environmental risks. Utilizing less toxic substances in manufacturing and lowering production temperatures are part of the plan. Concerns about the safety of emergency responders confronted with unidentifiable chemical spills originating from unmarked tanks and containers have been raised and answered. Color-coded warning systems have been put in place to instantly identify hazardous contents and dangerous levels of chemical cargo. The color placards are prominently displayed on the freight containers, rail cars, and trucks used in shipping. Blue tags signal poisonous and infectious chemicals. Red tags stand for flammable chemicals, and yellow tags represent radioactive materials. Other reforms and innovations no doubt lie ahead.

The biggest accidental chemical spill in United States history struck in Minot, North Dakota on January 18, 2002. In subzero weather, a Canadian Pacific train derailed and exploded at 2:30 a.m. Tanker cars full of anhydrous ammonia ruptured. One car shot 600 feet into the air, and another ripped in half and skated to a stop on the frozen Souris River. A noxious gas plume filled the air and 250,000 gallons of the poison were dumped on residential neighborhoods.

Several factors worsened the disaster. First, the freezing cold and absence of wind delayed the dissipation of the chemicals. Second and most significant, official notification and public warning stalled for many long hours. People were shocked awake by the loud blast and screeching train. They saw the whiteout of smoke and smelled ammonia fumes, but they didn't know what was happening or what to do. A power outage caused a blackout and snuffed out TV news. Anxious citizens turned on their battery-powered radios for breaking news and official instruction but the Emergency Alert System on the local station, KCJB, was down. In fact, listeners only heard canned, easy listening music on all six preprogrammed local radio stations. Without live reporting, affected residents were kept in the dark about the accident and its dangers.

Confusion and panic broke out, and people ran out into the street and into harm's way. Police phone lines and emergency radio lines were jammed with calls. Finally, the police commander sped to the home of the news director of KCJB, and woke him out of a sound sleep. The newsman drove through the toxic fog in the dead of night and announced the derailment on the air. Records show that, in spite of communication lapses, just one person died. Fifteen others were hospitalized, and a total of 1,600 sought medical care. Some of the victims were forced to evacuate for up to six weeks. And while not everyone would agree with the article that appeared in *Slate magazine*, it does share one version of the events of that fateful night (www.slate.com/id/2157395).

The drama of a chemical disaster usually hits the news with instant video feeds of the chaos, deaths, and injuries; but these acute effects are often overshadowed by slow developing, long-term ramifications. Chronic effects of chemical exposure have surfaced decades later when victims develop cancers and other illnesses. Cancer researchers have since tracked the broad and deeply serious harm caused by carcinogens released into the environment through these types of events and accidents.

In 1976, a pesticide plant explosion in Medea, Italy permeated the atmosphere with a cloud of dioxin gas that floated to nearby Seveso. A potent, cancer causing chemical, trichlorophenol, escaped from the ICMESA plant blanketing the densely populated city. Decades later, researchers studied breast cancer patients exposed to the dioxin release back in 1976. The Seveso women in the study all exhibited extremely high levels of the deadly carcinogen in their blood. The study results, published in 2002, concluded that a link to the ICMESA dioxin had been established.

Evidence has also shown that releases of dioxins into the environment cause severe harm immediately *and* long-term. Carcinogenic chemical spills that pollute water supplies have been shown to endanger large populations over time.

Complications can also arise from incomplete cleanups. In November 2005, a Petro Chemical plant explosion near the northeast border of China, in Jilin, dumped 100-tons of benzene into the Songhua River and tainted the water supply for millions. The lethal chemical absorbed into the water and cut the huge population off from the water supply it was dependent on. A $125,000 fine was levied against Petro Chemical, but the cleanup of the spill was not complete. Barrels of the poison are still being extracted by crews in 2011.

Delays in public warning have been shown to multiply the harm endured by disaster victims and environments. A scandal erupted on a pollution cover-up in East China in 2010. More than 60,000 innocent victims in the Fujian province were unknowingly exposed to two virulent waste tank leaks from the Zijin copper mine. The first gorged the Mianhuatan Reservoir with 2,403,965 gallons of copper waste. The Zijin Mining Group, China's leading gold and copper producer, failed to act immediately with public warnings. Mine officials waited a week to report the first leak. The second leak was traced to the number three tank after 132,086 gallons of toxins were expelled into the Tingjiang River. The mineral byproducts turned the water a ghostly blue and left it full of several thousand tons of rotting fish. In the scandal's wake, those held responsible were taken down by police and the government. Three Zijin executives were arrested, two environmental protection officials were suspended, and three government officials were fired.

Hydrocarbons are another type of chemical that can be a deadly poison over the long-term. Crude oil spills have blighted waterways and ravaged the land, devastating human populations and wildlife habitats with catastrophic effects of pollution. The largest accidental oil spill of all time happened when the BP Deepwater Horizon drilling rig exploded

50 miles off the coast of Louisiana in 2010, leaving a staggering legacy of pollution in the Gulf of Mexico. From April to July 2010, a leak from the ocean floor well spewed five million barrels of crude oil into the gulf waters—fouling the shores of four states.

While the Federal government downplayed the magnitude of the disaster, live video feeds of the sea floor gusher ran on the nightly news. Remote controlled subsea robots videoed the leak and sent the "spill cam" footage to TV broadcasters. Public outrage grew. The high pressures and cold temperatures of the deep sea environment posed difficulties in stopping the leak. A series of attempts to cap the wellhead failed, and the leak was finally stopped after an odyssey of 99 days.

This evidence shows that deep water drillers have pushed finite limits and taken big environmental risks. In hot pursuit of the wealth of oil and gas, they have ignored scientists' safety warnings and ventured farther from shore and ever deeper into the ocean's depths. In fact, BP had mapped a plan to drill down 18,000 feet in the near future. The stellar technological achievement is impressive, but it stands alone. It is not equaled by excellence in prevention, preparedness, and mitigation of oil spills. Experts agree, cooperation between government and private business interests will be necessary to strike a balance and surpass the singular quest for oil's black gold.

Not all oil well spills have been accidental. Unthinkable acts of sabotage are committed in wartime. During the Gulf war in 1991, a deliberate mega release of crude oil struck a punishing blow in Kuwait and polluted the Persian Gulf. An estimated 10 million barrels of toxic petroleum were dumped into the marine and coastal habitats. It was the largest spill in history, five times the size of the Deepwater

Toxic Chemical Releases

Horizon in 2010. The huge slick spread down the coast and into Saudi Arabia where it blackened the coastline and beaches. Over 30,000 water birds were killed and the ecosystem was badly damaged. Clean-up efforts were hampered by the ongoing military conflict. The fires set to 700 oil wells by fleeing Iraqi troops were later extinguished using explosive charges, but the global impact of the Iraqi attacks reached well beyond the Persian Gulf into the earth's atmosphere and ozone layer.

History shows that chemical disasters strike worldwide, pervading marine and land environments with destruction and pollution. The list includes chemical plant explosions, train derailments, oil well blowouts, tanker collisions and groundings, toxic waste leaks, and even pipeline sabotage. These sudden events wreak havoc on humans and wildlife, destroying homes, communities, and habitats. The impact extends to individual livelihoods and economies worldwide.

Below are action steps you can take to protect yourself and your household in the event of a toxic chemical release.

Before a Chemical Release

- ❑ Make a household or family plan.
- ❑ Locate a safe place to take cover, such as a basement or an interior room. Go to an upper floor if chemicals are on the ground.
- ❑ Take first aid classes and learn CPR.
- ❑ Be aware of local emergency response plans, spill control, and clean-up procedures and responses.
- ❑ Contact schools and your workplace for their emergency plans, notifications, and evacuation routes.
- ❑ Create emergency kits for home, school, work, and car.
- ❑ Put a change of clothing in your car or at work in case of chemical contamination.

- Store double black plastic garbage bags to dispose of contaminated clothing.
- Keep cash and change in emergency kits.
- Store canned food, water, and supplies.
- In first aid kit have essential prescription medications, spare eyeglasses
- Have plastic sheeting and duct tape for sealing up windows and vents.
- Learn about hazardous materials and chemicals.
- Check out nearby chemical plants, facilities, oil drilling operations, and factories for their emergency plans.
- Find safety and emergency information in utility bills and online.
- Check community calendars for educational emergency events.
- Attend neighborhood and community meetings and workshops.
- Register handicapped or disabled household or family members with a local emergency management agency.
- Know to limit exposure to the source of a chemical release.
- Be aware that chlorine gas is yellow-green in color, and stays low to the ground.
- Be aware that the chemical release could be invisible and odorless.
- Get information on health risks to children, the elderly, pregnant women, and adults.
- Be aware that a lot of people vomiting or lying on the ground may be reacting to toxic chemicals.
- Know that shortness of breath, tight chest, and coughing are often signs of toxic exposure.
- Know where to seek treatment by checking online for local hospitals or clinics.

Toxic Chemical Releases

- ❏ Use your cell phone to find emergency medical services.
- ❏ Recognize signs of exposure: skin reddening, blisters, and frostbite.
  - Know that red, burning, watery eyes, and blurry vision can be signs of exposure.
- ❏ Check on retirement home emergency plans and procedures.
- ❏ Check on apartment community emergency plan and emergency supplies.
- ❏ Check on local chemical warning systems, sirens, and emergency radio options.
- ❏ Teach the warning system signals to household members and children.
- ❏ Save the Emergency Broadcast Station on your radio memory panel.
- ❏ Plan evacuation routes; walk and drive alternate routes.
- ❏ Keep car tank filled with gas in case of evacuation.
- ❏ Find temporary shelter for pets through a veterinarian.
- ❏ Check on temporary lodging 10 to 50 miles away in case evacuation is required.
- ❏ Use your out-of-area contact person to synchronize messages between household and family members.

During a Chemical Release

- ✓ Know that hazardous chemicals may not be detected by sight, smell, or touch.
  - Check for burning eyes, nose, throat or coughing that can signal toxic exposure.
  - Check for shortness of breath and know that breathing problems could be signs of exposure.
  - Seek medical help as soon as possible.
- ✓ If you see a toxic cloud, or think toxic chemicals are present, immediately take shelter to limit exposure.

- ✓ Look on the ground for foamy or oily substances and avoid contact.
- ✓ Do not try to assist victims until authorities announce that it is safe.
- ✓ Cover nose and mouth with a cloth; take shallow breaths to lessen exposure.
- ✓ Stay uphill, upwind, and upstream from the disaster site.
- ✓ Limit the amount of time spent near the source of the chemical release.
- ✓ Get away from the hazardous site as quickly as possible.
- ✓ Shelter inside if you are at home, school, or work.
- ✓ Call 9-1-1 only in case of a life or death emergency.
- ✓ Be aware that chemicals dissipate over time.
- ✓ Stay inside until authorities announce that it is safe to come out.
- ✓ If you are driving in your car, close all windows tightly and turn off vents.
- ✓ Shut-off AC or car heater.
- ✓ Tune into public or radio alerts for information.
- ✓ If exposed to chlorine (yellow-green gas), wash off and call 9-1-1.
    - Remove contaminated clothing immediately. Cut it off, do not pull it over your head.
    - Seek treatment for chlorine poisoning at the nearest hospital.
    - Dispose of contaminated clothes, shoes, and contact lenses in double-sealed plastic bags.
    - Find a water source and clean entire body with soap and water.
    - Put on clean clothing and spare shoes from the emergency kit.

- Place clothing bags in garage or outside; minimize your exposure.
✓ If eyes are burning or you have blurry vision, rinse eyes with water for 10 to 15 minutes.
✓ Close off rooms not used much, storage, guest rooms, laundry, etc.
✓ Keep pets inside if possible.
✓ Shut and lock all doors and windows.
✓ Seal windows, vents, and air ducts with duct tape and plastic sheeting.
✓ Close fireplace and wood stove dampers; seal off furnaces.
✓ Duct tape stove and dryer vents, or use tin foil, wax paper, or plastic sheeting to block the openings.
✓ Shut-off ventilation systems, heating and cooling.
✓ If you have a basement area or cellar, go there and take cover or go to an upper floor if chemicals are on the ground.
✓ Stay behind concrete or glass to shield from harmful chemicals.
✓ Monitor Emergency Broadcast System and social media for updates and instruction.
✓ Remain inside until the all clear is given by authorities.

After a Chemical Release

❑ Follow authorities' directions to stay inside at home, school, or work.
❑ Be aware that chemicals may not be detected by sight or smell.
  - Know to minimize exposure to toxic chemicals.
❑ Continue to monitor social media, radio, and news feeds.
❑ Help others as possible: handicapped, children, and elderly first.

- ❑ Avoid eating exposed fruits and vegetables that may be contaminated.
  - Do not eat any crops not yet harvested.
  - Wash and peel any fruits or vegetables stored inside.
- ❑ Bring pets inside if possible or contain them in a garage if exposed.
- ❑ Avoid stirring up or breathing in dust as it may be toxic.
- ❑ Provide as much shelter for livestock as possible, especially those producing milk.
- ❑ Give all animals previously stored feed and water.
- ❑ Store previously harvested garden crops inside.
- ❑ Do not get in the way of emergency responders cleaning up the spill.
- ❑ Use food, water, and supplies from your pre-assembled emergency kits.
- ❑ Call, text, or use social media to contact household and family members to report your situation.
- ❑ If told to evacuate, follow directions of authorities, relocate to official safe area.
  - Be aware it is important to quickly put distance between you and the hazardous spill.
  - Take emergency kit and stored food, water, and supplies with you.
  - Do not deviate from safe routes that authorities give, do not take short cuts.
  - Make contact with your out-of-area contact person.

POWER OUTAGES

In the modern world, the supply of electrical energy is in incessant global demand. Nations and populations are dependent on electric power for the basic necessities of everyday life. Essential activities like washing clothes, cooking food, using computers, and communicating on cell phones all rely on power. Lighting, heating, refrigeration, and air conditioning shut down when the power goes out. Public drinking supplies are cut off when water cannot be pumped from dams and reservoirs, and irrigation water for farmland crops and livestock dry up as well.

Electrical energy also serves hospitals, nuclear plants, transportation systems, businesses, banks, the military, and government. Power outages can pose only a few hours of inconvenience, but they can also be life changing and cascade into disasters. Local blackouts and larger regional grid outages have plunged cities, states, and countries into darkness for elongated periods of time. Lives and economies have been endangered by a loss of power.

Debilitating power outages have been part of the history of natural and man-made disasters. It has been shown time and again that when the flow of power stops, regions come to a standstill and go into crisis mode. This massive disruption suspends normal activities and routine daily commerce. All at once, millions of people come unhinged by the gridlock. High rise elevators stall, and workers sprint down stairwells to flee office buildings. Public transit stops dead in its tracks. Traffic signals go dark. Vehicles get tangled in paralyzing traffic jams and commuters are stranded. Airline passengers face canceled flights. Citizens and travelers are trapped in the dark and cut off without cell phone transmission. Hospitals struggle to provide patient care and keep surgeries, emergency rooms, and maternity wards on track.

People on the streets face physical dangers as well. Downed power lines and live wires pose threats of electrical shock. Gas powered generators used as electrical backups have also jeopardized lives with their poisonous carbon monoxide emissions. When heat and air conditioning systems shut down, extreme winter cold and summer heat have produced disabling or fatal cases of hypothermia, dehydration, or heat stroke. The health of the economy has been put at risk too. Downed computer networks cripple businesses and financial institutions, and cause huge financial losses.

The causes of power outages and blackouts are prolific and well documented. Violent seasonal storms and a host of natural disasters have wiped out electrical transmission lines, and wrecked generators and nuclear power plants. Summer thunderstorms have hurled lightning bolts that seared power poles and exploded electrical components. Blustering winter blizzards iced tree limbs and snapped electrical lines. The turbo winds and rains of hurricanes, cyclones, and typhoons have obliterated entire electric grids and robbed wide regions of their vital electrical juice.

The world watched in 2005 as Hurricane Katrina drowned New Orleans in flood waters that snuffed out the city's power. Elsewhere, mighty earthquakes shook and tumbled the land, ruptured gas lines and spread roaring fires that cremated power transmitters. In 2011, the uproar of a magnitude 9.0 quake rocked the east coast of Japan and launched a jet speed tsunami that leveled port cities. It uprooted trees and power lines like twigs, and trounced generators and nuclear reactors in a matter of minutes. The sheer force of these raging natural disasters and their incomprehensible damage has riveted global attention. Blackouts have been just one ingredient in this complex recipe of destruction and upheaval.

Major electrical blackouts have joined history's roster

of both natural and man-made disasters. *Wired Magazine* reported a huge power outage that hit North America during the winter of 1998 and lasted for over a month. Four Canadian provinces and four northeastern United States were walloped by ice storms that took out 1,000 transmission towers and 35,000 utility poles. Over five million people suffered without electrical service for 33 bone-chilling days, and 100,000 victims had to evacuate their homes and seek relief in shelters. The event dragged on from January 5, 1998 to February 8, 1998. Forty-five people paid with their lives, and insurance costs burgeoned to $1.2 billion dollars. In Malaysia in 1992, an earlier event had affected a much larger population. Eighteen million people lost power in nine of the country's 13 states due to a lightning strike. Silicon Island manufacturers were shut down, and trading on the national stock exchange was suspended. In just 48-hours, business losses escalated to $220 million.

Man-made disasters can cause power outages as well, and equipment failure has resulted in serious damage to high-demand electrical networks. In one instance in 1981, a blockbuster power outage in Mexico started with three generator failures and left 39 million people without electrical service. The inhabitants of Mexico City, along with 15 states, were victimized by the cascading accident. Lights went out all over the country, affecting 60 percent of the Mexican population. Gridlock ensued, while a gigantic traffic jam held two million vehicles prisoner, and 40,000 commuters were stuck on subways.

In 2010 and 2011 in Pakistan, a population of 165 million was plagued by daily power outages from outdated equipment and lack of fuel. The valued United States ally has endured the insurgency of the Taliban and still managed to grow its economy, but in recent years, commerce and capital have increasingly been impacted by electrical shortfalls. A battle over wattage has since ensued. Every day 16,000 megawatts are required to power the country, but only 10,000 megawatts can be supplied by Pakistan's antiquated and fuel deprived power plants.

The once abundant natural resources of gas and oil have petered out. Shortfalls of these essential fuel sources have curbed production and the churning of power, while electric service has been meager. The supply of power to households, dams, businesses, and government has not met demand in many years. Water supply shortages have also added to the mix.

These shrunken energy resources and increasing electrical power needs have pulled Pakistan down into the dark, depleting the once promising economy. According to *Pakistan Today*, the country's crucial exports have dropped by 50 percent due to the struggle to keep the lights on, run factories, and pump water. Broken down power plants have ground cities to a halt with daily power outages lasting 10 to 20 hours. Industry and farming have curtailed operations too, and the power crisis has spurred violent demonstrations in Lahore and Karachi. A 2010 *McClatchy Newspapers* piece described an angry mob that broke into a power riot against the Pakistan Electric Power Company (PEPCO) in the streets of Lahore, leaving one person dead. The government-run company was unable to broker a solution to the conflict.

In an effort to make due with a short power supply, Pakistan resorted to government regulated energy conservation, and scheduled outages became the norm. In rural areas, farmers were hit hard by the power cutbacks; unable to run their electric water pumps to irrigate crops and fields. Ordinary people were required to make drastic lifestyle changes. Household appliances could not be run and laundry had to wait. Lights were out and children's homework was put on hold. One implementation known as "dual load shedding" cut supplies of both electricity and natural gas. Transportation was slowed to a snail's pace when the two million vehicles fueled by natural gas ran little or sat idle.

Power sharing was another part of the conservation plan. Designated portions of Karachi, Lahore and other cities took turns waiting in line to use their electrical allotments. The Punjab province, home to half the population, banned energy hungry neon signs, billboards, and exterior building lights; and shut off streetlights and fountains. Relief from the constant 100-degree temperatures diminished due to air conditioning cut backs in hospitals, banks, shops, malls, factories, and government offices. Pakistan's custom of nighttime shopping was curtailed when lights went out in malls and shops after sunset. Wedding celebrations that once went on past midnight were ordered to end earlier. Clocks were set an hour ahead, and shorter workweeks were mandated.

The government's conservation plan met strong resistance. *National Geographic* reported on the civil unrest caused by the planned outages in May 2010. Screaming demonstrators burned tires in the streets of Karachi, rioting against the Karachi Electric Supply Corporation (KESC). The stones and bottles hurled by enraged civilians were no match for police batons and tear gas. In 2011, unannounced power outages of 12 hours or more spiked tempers and roused more protests. Pakistan's most viable export was all but halted when textile factories lost their exemption and were put on the power outage schedule. Plants closed down three days a week.

Critics have denounced the measures as being too little, too late, and found the energy conservation approach and the lifestyle mandates ineffective. Economists from the Karachi-based Collective for Social Research take a less than positive view of Pakistan's energy future; saying that time is needed to build more hydroelectric power plants, erect windmills, and excavate mines. They maintain that crucial billions of dollars are needed to begin recovery even though the heavily indebted nation faces financial resource shortages along with its natural resource shortages. All sides agree that there is no quick solution for Pakistan, instead anticipating that it will take many, many years to fully recover.

Other large populations have suffered through major blackouts that have recurred over the years. In Brazil, some electric grid power shutdowns were originally attributed to natural causes, although later were discovered to be of man-made origin. Major drama struck the nation multiple times for over a decade, from 1999 to 2011. The continuous outages have forced hundreds of millions of citizens into the dark. A lightning strike on a Sao Paulo substation in 1999 shorted power to 97 million people. In January 2005, Rio de Janeiro and two other cities lost power; affecting tens of thousands of people. In 2007, in the state of Espirito Santo, three million Brazilian citizens struggled through a major blackout for two days.

In 2009, heavy storms reportedly shut down power to half of the country in the nation's worst outage yet. Brazil is the world's second largest hydroelectric producer, but all went black when transmission lines from the Itaipu Dam stopped working. Business, commerce, and transport floundered and then went into lock down. Subways and elevators froze up, streetlights and traffic lights were extinguished. Brazilian government representatives and utility company spokesmen cited the stormy weather as the cause of the incident and publically dismissed any possibility of espionage.

The National Space Research Institute went public too, refuting the claim that the storms had caused such an enormous disruption, while researchers said evidence and probability of weather-related causes were absent. Later revelations followed, pinpointing the cause of the disaster on cyber-attacks carried out by distant computer hackers. Confirmation of the source of the Brazil blackouts appeared in print in an article published by the *Foreign Policy Journal* on November 15, 2009. It reported that all of the power outages may have been due to cyber espionage of unknown foreign origin.

An interview in *Wired Magazine* featured Richard Clark, former special advisor on cyber security to United States President George W. Bush. Mr. Clark flatly stated that computer hackers had been successful at halting power in Brazil. The concept, unfortunately, was not a new one. Years earlier, in 2007, United States CIA chief security officer Tom Donahue publicly admitted in a New Orleans speech that hackers were successful in breaching foreign computer systems to cut off power to multiple cities. These candid statements were perceived as a warning to private utility companies to spur them into action in the face of impending security threats.

Security professionals have agreed that the time is now for Brazil to resolve its vulnerability to further attacks. In a 2009 *Foreign Policy Journal* article, security specialist and consultant Michael MyIrea voiced concerns over Brazil's inefficient and outdated electrical power grid and security deficient computer systems. He pointed out that the official government website had been vulnerable in 2008 when it was penetrated by cyber hackers. Three thousand employees were robbed of access to their system for 24-hours. The $350 million ransom demand that followed the break-in was not paid, but there was a high cost in compromised data and lost time. Wrenching the system out of the hands of the hackers took seven frenzied days of code cracking.

According to MyIrea, Brazil's computer network is only one part of the infrastructure at risk. He says the entire energy infrastructure and nation's economy are also seriously endangered by escalating cyber intrusions in the near future. In his opinion, government legislation and considerable capital investment are necessary to beef up security, make transmission upgrades and improve load management.

In 2010, yet another blackout made its mark on Brazil's repeating history of electrical outages and power was chopped off in seven states. The event was officially attributed to dead transmission lines at an electrical substation. In 2011, more power outages reportedly shook up the grid and toppled power. The country's aging infrastructure and lax security stand to be tested by two eminent, high-profile sporting events that will draw millions of athletes, fans, locals, and visitors. The nation will host soccer's World Cup in 2014, and serve as the venue for the Summer Olympic Games in Rio de Janeiro in 2016.

It is not only second-world countries that fight the battle of electrical outages. The biggest blackout in United States history brought New York City to a grinding halt during a 90 degree heat wave in August 2003. The massive outage was later confirmed to be a cyber-attack. According to *CBS News*, nine nuclear plant reactors were without power over a broad span of more than 9,300 square miles in eight northeastern states and throughout southeast Canada.

Fifty million people in the United States were without lights, water, air conditioning, or public transit. Rush hour subways and trains stopped running, and weary, overheated workers walked miles on foot to get home or to work. Hospitals ran on backup generators, while airports grounded planes at Kennedy, La Guardia, Newark, Cleveland, Toronto, and Ottawa while passengers waited. The Detroit-Windsor

Tunnel denied passage to its daily capacity of 27,000 cars and trucks, leaving commuters stuck. A total of 100 power plants had abruptly ceased electrical transmission.

From its base in Bethesda, Maryland, the Nuclear Regulatory Commission concisely cited loss of offsite power as the catalyst for the disaster. Canadian authorities blamed a lightning strike on a power plant near Niagara Falls for the outage. An article in *Scientific American* fleshed out a description of the power meltdown and reported high voltage lines had overheated in north Ohio, colliding with overgrown treetops causing a domino shutdown effect. For an unknown reason at the time, the utility company, First Energy Corporation, was not alerted by its automated alarm system, and so the shutdowns spread unchecked. Eleven human lives were lost, and the economic cost was $6 billion dollars.

A thorough investigation of the 2003 blackout commenced and brought changes in the energy industry with heightened standards and regulations. After three months of work, the United States-Canada Power System Outage Task Force concluded that equipment failure and human error unleashed the event. The Energy Policy Act of 2005 was passed in Congress requiring the Federal Energy Regulatory Commission (FERC) to strengthen its rules. Forty-six recommendations for reducing the risk of large blackouts were put in place.

The FERC was also required to set and enforce 96 new mandatory reliability standards, called trees, training, and tools. Trees had to be trimmed away from power lines, workers needed increased crisis training, and grid operating systems had to be capable of surviving big power failures. Violators would pay hefty fines of up to $1 million per day. Carnegie Mellon University researchers reviewed data from 1984–2006 and found that blackouts for populations of

50,000 or more remained constant at twelve per year, despite new regulations.

On May 31, 2008, the cause of the 9,300 mile blackout over the northeastern United States and Canada in 2003 finally came to light and it had nothing to do with overgrown trees or lightning strikes. *The National Journal* published a definitive statement from Tim Bennett, former president of the Cyber Security Industry Alliance. He disclosed that United States intelligence sources utilized forensic analysis that traced the massive power outage back to Chinese computer hackers of the People's Liberation Army (PLA). The evidence also confirmed how First Energy's power control network had been infected with a computer virus that disabled the company's alarm system and silenced the automatic alert.

Jim Lewis, director of the Center for Strategic and International Studies heads the committee that recently compiled and delivered an in-depth report on cyber security to United States President Barack Obama. Mr. Lewis reiterated the concerns of other experts indicating that the possibilities for espionage are boundless in a cyber-connected world, with computer databases and power networks susceptible to compromise and disruption every day. To illuminate the weakness of security, he shared multiple stories of cyber hackers wreaking havoc on the computer-run electrical grid systems of many nations and their governments including the United States. The growing frequency of cyber intrusions spotlight a glaring lack of protection in the national infrastructure and raise the need for immediate action on energy security.

Private business composed of public power providers, corporate giants, and financial companies align on criticisms of the United States government in this regard. Good news has followed from the FBI and the Department of Homeland Security (DHS). A confidential forum has been established allowing businesses to freely disclose their vulnerabilities and receive customized security assistance from the government's public sector. As the documented evidence suggests, the costs of poor security in an ominous cyber world are unacceptably high.

The National Security Agency (NSA) took defensive action to prevent security breaches and infrastructure disruptions and created Cyber Attack Protection in 2010. The surveillance system was brought forth from the lab and dubbed "Perfect Citizen." It was programmed to perform functions such as checking threats against electrical networks and watching over nuclear power plants and transport systems. When *The Wall Street Journal* leaked the news of "Perfect Citizen" in July 2010, it struck a nerve. Consumer advocates and privacy watchdogs fighting for the rights of ordinary citizens rose up in protest. In the meantime, while "Perfect Citizen" minds the store, blackouts continue to befall communities and nations.

In the face of the mounting concerns more action is being taken, and a trillion dollars will be spent to launch a 20-year expansion of the utility industry. The North American Electrical Reliability Corporation (NERC) and the Department of Energy (DOE) have partnered to study the implications of simultaneous power outages that could impact millions of residences, businesses, banks, government, and the military. The project will focus on protecting the electrical grid from widespread and long-term power interruptions including bursts of the sun's radiation called solar flares. Advanced automated controls will enable grid managers to isolate susceptible parts of the network and prevent power losses from solar flare strikes. The new technology will speed blackout recovery efforts as well. Smart grid technology, renewable energy transmission, and green energy technology will all be developed and implemented to safeguard the crucial power network.

As we have illustrated, the power grid keeps the world turning. The importance of electrical energy as a resource cannot be overstated. It runs the computers that serve the grid and powers homes, businesses, banks, hospitals, and the government. Computers are cyber-connected and Internet accessible; they switch on lights, heating, gas pumps, and water supplies. Blackouts from both natural and manmade causes have impacted lives and economies in cities and regions worldwide. Extreme electrical shutdowns have caused injuries and death while also racking up huge dollar costs, property damages, and economic losses.

Important Information to Report Regarding an Outage:
- Name and address.
- Time and date of outage.
- If lights are flickering or dim.
- If other lights are out on homes or businesses nearby.
- Note any loud noise before the outage.
- Note downed wires or tree limbs on wires.

Any fallen power lines should be considered "live." If you see a power line on the ground, do not touch it. If the power line is touching someone—stay away. Electricity is invisible. If you touch that person you could become a victim too. Call the power company to report it along with the information above. If a power line falls on your car, don't get out. Stay inside and wait for emergency responders' help.

Below are action steps to protect you and your household in the event of an electrical outage.

Before a Power Outage

- ☐ Know a power blackout will be sudden and affect infrastructure.
- ☐ Plan alternate driving and walking routes, and transportation.
- ☐ Be aware that the gasoline supply may be limited.
  - Know service stations rely on electricity to pump gas.
- ☐ Keep gas tanks of vehicles at least half full.
- ☐ Locate the electrical panel, test and label circuit breaker switches.
- ☐ Check with neighbors to find out who owns a generator.
- ☐ Know not to run a generator inside your home as it can emit poisonous carbon monoxide.
- ☐ Consider buying a generator for backup power.
- ☐ Have a portable, battery-powered radio on hand.
- ☐ Set cell phones to public alerts and social media sites for updates.
- ☐ Tape extra batteries to outside of radio or get crank radio and crank cell phone chargers.
- ☐ Include a flashlight for each household member and chargers or extra batteries.
- ☐ Keep warm blanket, clothes, and shoes in car trunk in case you get wet and cold.
- ☐ Store water and canned or freeze-dried food.
  - Learn about food safety and storage.
  - Get a digital thermometer for testing food.
  - Know that a half full refrigerator can keep food safely for 24 hours.
  - Know a full refrigerator keeps food safely for 48 hours.
- ☐ Take a first aid class from the Red Cross, community center, or fire station.
  - Learn Cardiac Pulmonary Resuscitation (CPR).

- Learn the dangers of hypothermia and how to avoid or treat.
- Learn signs of heatstroke and how to avoid or treat.

❏ Know carbon monoxide (CO) fumes can be poisonous.
  - Be aware that CO is an odorless, invisible gas emitted from gas appliances, oil, wood, and coal heat.
  - Know flu-like symptoms can mean CO poisoning, and what actions to take.

❏ Install battery operated CO detectors near CO sources such as gas stove, fireplace, etc.
  - Check batteries twice a year, replace device every five years.

❏ Be aware that cordless phones need electricity to operate.

❏ Know that if transmission towers are down, cell phones may be out of service.

❏ Know how to use Twitter or other social media sites for help.

❏ Be prepared with charged cell phones.
  - Know USB ports are often needed to connect to chargers.
  - Upgrade cell phones; buy chargers and connector cords.

❏ Learn to use GPS mapping systems.

❏ Add disaster alert applications to cell phones.
  - Check out medical help apps on your phone, tablet, or other mobile device.
  - Tune into early disaster alerts via cell phone as soon as possible.

❏ Locate community centers and online bulletin boards for emergency information.

❏ Go to a nearby fire station to check HAM radio communications.

- ❑ Get information on utility plant failures, grid outages, and instructions via online crisis response sites.

During a Power Outage

- ✓ Don't try to drive unnecessarily.
- ✓ If driving, watch out for downed or falling power lines.
- ✓ Be aware that contact with power lines could cause electrocution.
- ✓ If a power line falls on your car, stay inside and call 9-1-1.
  - Warn those nearby not to touch car, ask them to call 9-1-1.
- ✓ If car catches on fire, leave by opening the door and jumping free.
- ✓ To avoid electric shock, keep both feet on the ground and shuffle 50 feet away until clear.
- ✓ Do not risk shock by assisting passengers, have them jump clear of car.
- ✓ Be aware of dangers of electrical shock and first aid steps.
- ✓ Know electrical current could pass through you if you touch a victim of electrical shock.
- ✓ Turn off the source of electricity if possible.
- ✓ Use nonconductive wood, plastic, or cardboard to move the electrical source away from the victim.
- ✓ Take victim's pulse, check breathing, and perform CPR if capable.
  - Lay or sit victim down, knees elevated if in shock, pale, or faint.
  - Do not remove burned clothes or touch burns.
  - Be aware that internal burns may be present.
  - Get medical help immediately at a clinic, hospital, or fire station.

- ✓ If outside in cold weather, put on heavy coat or blanket from car trunk.
- ✓ Know dangers of low body temperature and hypothermia and how to treat.
- ✓ Avoid immersion in water or puddles, and wear high rubber boots.
- ✓ If wet, immediately change into dry clothes, shoes, and hat.
- ✓ If going outside in hot weather, layer in light, loose clothing.
  - Stay in the shade as much as possible.
  - Wear protection such as a broad-brimmed hat.
- ✓ Adjust work hours for coolest times of day, evening.
- ✓ Get inside a mall or other building with air conditioning or a backup generator.
- ✓ Know temperature of 106 degrees Fahrenheit or more can mean heatstroke.
  - Watch for signs of reddened skin, no sweating, dizziness, loss of concentration.
  - Sit or lie down in the shade if heat stroke symptoms are present.
  - Find refuge in a shelter or medical facility if in danger of heat stroke. Check social media sites and public alerts.
- ✓ Know that 9-1-1 circuits will be overloaded.
- ✓ Be aware that most heaters, air conditioning, and fans will not work without electricity.
- ✓ Leave one light switch on to signal when power returns.
- ✓ Unplug appliances and electronics to avoid a power surge when power returns.
- ✓ Use a flashlight instead of candles to avoid fire danger.
- ✓ Tune in to social media or public emergency alerts for information.

Power Outages

- ✓ Stay tuned to radio or cell phone for alerts on power outages and instructions.
- ✓ Be alert for terrorist threat notifications.
- ✓ Stay alert for changing conditions, traffic, and infrastructure shutdowns.
- ✓ Pack perishable food in a small cooler with ice to have it keep longer.
- ✓ Don't open your freezer or refrigerator unnecessarily.
  - Mark the date and time when power is out, post on freezer and refrigerator doors.
  - Eat perishable foods first, before they spoil.
  - Be aware that two hours without power could spoil milk and dairy products.
  - Know that meat, fish, eggs, and leftovers may be unsafe after two hours without power.
  - Use food thermometer to check food for temperature.
  - Discard foods that are spoiled or unsafe, or over 40 degrees Fahrenheit.
- ✓ Be aware that water may be limited as supply needs electricity to pump.
  - Be aware of water shortages and manage what you have for maximum use.
- ✓ Drink one gallon of water per day, or eight ounces every 15 minutes.
  - Know it is important to stay hydrated, drink water.
  - Avoid dehydration from alcohol and caffeine. Limit salty foods.
  - Drink bottled or treated water; boil water if necessary.
  - Fill bathtub and sinks with uncontaminated tap water for emergency drinking supply.
- ✓ Be aware that a generator can emit poisonous carbon monoxide (CO) fumes.

- ✓ Don't run a generator or barbeque in your home, garage, or enclosed porch or near doors, windows, or vents.
- ✓ Do not plug generator directly into electrical system to avoid power line surge.
- ✓ Know that dizziness, nausea, vomiting, and fatigue are all signs of CO poisoning.
- ✓ If cold at home, avoid hypothermia by layering clothes and wrapping yourself in blankets.
- ✓ When power returns, do not overload system by plugging all devices back in all at once.
- ✓ Don't drive if you can avoid it, due to downed power lines and traffic jams.

After a Power Outage

- ❑ Limit driving.
- ❑ Be aware of possible traffic gridlock and public transportation stalls.
- ❑ Avoid downed power lines if outside, report to utility company, police.
- ❑ If wet or cold, immediately change into dry clothes and shoes.
- ❑ If near heavy equipment, beware of sudden return of power that might restart it.
- ❑ Restock water bottles, food, supplies, and batteries in case power goes off again.
- ❑ Continue to use flashlights and battery powered lanterns for light.
- ❑ Do not light candles due to fire danger.
- ❑ Stay tuned to radio local emergency broadcast, get information and instructions.
- ❑ Treat your injuries first, next check on household or family members and children; render first aid.

Power Outages

- ☐ Watch for heat or cold related illnesses like heat stroke or hypothermia.
- ☐ Check refrigerated and frozen foods for spoilage and discard if necessary.
- ☐ Cook or consume only safe foods.
- ☐ Check in with relatives, neighbors, and out-of-area contact person for updates on the situation.
- ☐ Check on elderly, disabled, ill, or pregnant neighbors.
- ☐ Check on pets, livestock.
- ☐ Be aware that other outages could follow, and monitor public alerts.

Communications in a Disaster

In an emergency, communications will be altered. Terror-filled moments, hours, and days may be spent trying to reach loved ones. There are many ways to safeguard yourself and your family inside and outside of affected disaster areas by utilizing up-to-date communications applications. Today's plethora of cell phone applications for smart phones and Android phones provides pre-disaster planning tools you can carry in your pocket. By using sites such as Twitter, Facebook, and Google you can tune into rapid recovery response web information that is sent out from these sites in mere minutes to hours after a disaster.

If you can say it in 140 characters or less, then you can get your message out on Twitter even when phone lines are down. This could be crucial if you want to communicate in a disaster. You should invest time now learning how to use social media tools before a disaster strikes. According to the Internet site Mashable, after the March 11, 2011 Japan earthquake and tsunami, 1,200 tweets per minute were sent from Tokyo. Twitter also reported record tweets that day of over 176 million. The day after the earthquake and tsunami over 100,000 Twitter accounts were added by new users.

In May 2011, the Center for Disease Control (CDC) launched a warning of an impending zombie attack via their blog and Twitter. Residents of Japan in the affected area of the nuclear fallout were worried that they could become zombie-like from the radiation. It was a legitimate warning that resulted in many inquiries to the CDC. How the CDC dealt with this unprecedented scenario paved the way for organizations like FEMA to accept the use of social media to communicate disaster information in real-time. The result was a spike of over 30,000 hits to the CDC website when the news broke. Residents were encouraged to follow the same

263

protocol as if dealing with any other disaster (http://www.bt.cdc.gov/socialmedia/zombies_blog.asp). Regardless of the disaster, online and social media tools are excellent resources to access information and get necessary help.

Setting up an account ahead of a disaster may ensure your ability to login to this site in a disaster. It would also be a good idea to look online at some of the Twitter logs and other blogs before an emergency to understand this method of communicating. In a disaster, Twitter users have tweeted thousands of messages from all over the world using hashtags to connect on trending topics. Understanding the use of hashtags could be crucial to you in a disaster. From Japan to Chile, hashtags like #earthquakeChile and #tsunamiJapan have connected people in and out of the disaster affected area. A way to get familiar with content and daily updates on Twitter can be found on FEMA's Twitter page (see @FEMA on Twitter).

Blogs are another way to get crucial information out before, during, and after a disaster. Blogs are web logs of commentary and news. There are numerous blogs dedicated to emergency information that even include early warnings covering current weather and disaster related topics. One of the best sources to read about emergency services in blog format is online at Clark Regional Emergency Services Agency (http://cresa911.blogspot.com).

United States FEMA Administrator, Craig Fugate, has championed social media as a rapidly growing tool for two-way communication from emergency responders to the public in the event of a disaster. As of May 6, 2011, Fugate set a standard to include social media in emergency response planning by FEMA. You can follow Fugate and others in the newest conversations about social media by tracking them on

Twitter. For example, to access Social Media in Emergency Management, use #smem. To get information on the Red Cross, use #howihelp. If you are a Spanish speaker, check out the FEMA preparedness and disaster assistance Spanish language site (www.listo.gov).

You can also connect to people all over the world through HAM radio clubs. Local chapters offer training and licensing. Most importantly, HAM radios have been connecting people all over the world for decades. It is said to be the most reliable worldwide channel of communication in a disaster. Radio operators help restore communications in all major disasters and bring relief efforts to those in need. Go online for more details on how you can train for a HAM radio license in your area (http://ares.org).

The world has watched powerful natural disasters bring devastation to thousands of people in mere minutes. The world has also reacted with humanitarian efforts that have produced a whole new way to respond in a disaster for individuals, businesses, governments, and volunteers. This effort is called crowd sourcing. The Sahana Software Foundation website (http://sahanafoundation.org) shines a light on how this tool has been used after major earthquakes and tsunamis to create a channel between volunteers and emergency workers.

The use of crowd sourcing in disasters has forever changed how people see themselves as part of relief efforts—no matter where they are in the world. From countries all over the world, volunteers can aid in the design of maps via cloud computing for use by workers on the ground complete with language translation features. Humanitarian aid can be collected and disbursed with today's web technology. Search and rescue teams can get ground reports established through cooperation with telecommunications companies and businesses that have supplied software to help organize response efforts of volunteers.

This advanced technology has empowered people worldwide to give freely of their skills and contribute to disaster relief. Another place where you can read about the efforts of hundreds of volunteers responding to a worldwide disaster is on Ushahidi (which means "testimony "in Swahili). Read about volunteer mapping efforts in the Kenyan post-election crisis of 2008 (http://www.ushahidi.com). This army of volunteers can communicate their humanitarian goals and share disaster relief efforts with worldwide city responders. This interoperability has proved effective in the cities of New York and Los Angeles and with the private companies of IBM and Google. It's also gained support from the Red Cross and other first response agencies.

All of these technological advances mean that your phone can do just about anything to help you in a disaster. Free content from medical providers can guide you through splinting a limb to minor medical operations. One app can even dial your phone for you if you are caught and can only access one finger. Other phone apps have multi-language support so you can say "Emergency" in French, German, Spanish, or Italian. An application called the POM Alert instantly notifies you as disasters happen specific to your real-time location by combining information from FEMA, Homeland Security, and the National Weather Service. The Department of Homeland Security has a Twitter account you can sign up to follow, @NTASAlerts, to be notified of a disaster via Twitter, Facebook, RSS feed, or from their blog page. Once you receive an alert you can put your own emergency plan into action as needed and connect with your household members as planned.

In the resource guide that follows, we will provide a list of known applications that can do everything from alerting you to impending natural disasters to converting your phone into a flashlight, alarm, or emergency radio. The main concern with phones, however, is how long you can use your phone if there is no power. There are solar powered chargers that you can purchase for your phone, which will work if there is sunshine. There are also hand crank phone chargers for sale and you can purchase these through the Red Cross store and through AAA offices. They typically cost $24.99, and come with multiple phone jacks to fit any phone. In many cases, the crank mechanism often doubles as a flashlight. We recommend that you test this before a disaster strikes.

Emergency responders are trained to look at victim's cell phones for information in case of emergency (ICE). Most cell phones have a place for you to enter basic information about your health and any medications that you may be taking. Emergency information apps can keep your current medical conditions, surgical history, emergency contacts, and a mobile medical notebook for less than $3.00. Apps from places like WebMD are free and provide a symptom checker, first aid essentials, and more. ICE applications are available that can even "talk" for you if you are incapacitated. Also, explore Family Applications with ICE which can store up to eight profiles.

Volumes of maps are also available for download as a preparedness step. Any emergency plan should include a meeting place if you are separated from your household. MyMap at Google has an easy, fun, and stress-free tutorial for making your own map if you create it before disaster strikes. You can share it with household members and your out-of-area contact person. You can go public to share your map on your mobile browser with your neighborhood or community.

Free apps also exist as navigation tools that utilize over 10,000 traffic cameras to show weather, accidents, and other events that can affect your commute. *The Weather Channel* is one of the top content providers of information for phone apps used by consumers. Weather-related news for mobile phones is one of the most popular forms of downloaded content on smart phones with over 30 million cumulative downloads. Utilizing your phone and social media may be the best resource for you in a disaster to reach out to household members.

Mobile phone carriers are now using new technology to push out emergency alerts to mobile phones as part of a new service called Personal Localized Alerting Network (PLAN). This text message system will geographically target mobile phones with fast, useful, and potentially life-saving information. New phones already have the PLAN chip and some older phones may access this alerting system through a software upgrade. We have witnessed the communication power of smart phones and Twitter in 2011 with the volcanic eruption in Iceland, the earthquake and tsunami in Japan, and the political upheaval in Egypt and Libya. The fact that these devices—with their own batteries and Internet connections—can work even when landline phone service is down has been lifesaving.

Using Communications Before a Disaster

- ❑ Sign up for a Google account so you can use the Mapping tool to create your own evacuation plans that you can then share with household or family members (https://www.google.com/accounts/NewAccount).
    - Set up Google Real Time Alerts (www.google.com) to follow the most up-to-date news on the web, such as earthquake alerts, and emergency response.

Communications in a Disaster

- See the critical information available worldwide to help coordinate relief efforts in Haiti, Chile, Japan, and other current disaster-affected areas (http://www.google.com/crisisresponse) and see how communities are being drawn together through social media after a disaster strikes (http://rebuildjoplin.org).
- ❏ Read how to use Twitter (http://support.twitter.com) to learn how to create messages, search for topics, and find people.
  - Read how to get and send Twitter messages without signing up for Twitter (http://support.twitter.com/articles/218610-new-fast-follow).
  - Create a Twitter List of people you want to follow in a disaster and save them using a group feature for quick access (http://support.twitter.com).
- ❏ Go online (www.sm4em.org) for centralized reporting by social media and the world of emergency services. You can also access channels to comment via Twitter on real-time advances in social media and emergency management.
- ❏ See how worldwide efforts are bringing people together to render aid through open data technology (www.crisiscommons.org).
- ❏ Read about a non-profit that uses global volunteers, online tools, and multiple social networking sites to aid in global disasters (http://www.humanityroad.org/Home.htm).
- ❏ Read why the first 24-hours make the biggest difference for you in a disaster (http://challenge.gov/challenges/87/submissions/1085-the-303-plan-absolutely-everybody-in-the-whole-wide-world).
- ❏ Host your own conversation online with friends and family to discuss disaster planning, evacuation

plans, or important wishes before a disaster (http://www.talkshoe.com/talkshoe/web/main.jsp?pushNav=1&cmd=home).
- ❑ Learn how to compile all of your social media contacts (Facebook, Twitter, LinkedIn, Flickr, etc.) on one page (http://www.tweetdeck.com).
- ❑ Read about the huge army of volunteers who came together after the New Zealand earthquake in 2011 to help each other, and how they managed it all using a phone app (http://geoop.posterous.com/volunteer-army-of-students-uses-geoop-to-help).
- ❑ Set up a Facebook group so that in an emergency you can post your whereabouts privately to your family and friends (http://www.facebook.com/groups).
- ❑ Sign up to access disaster news reports from your phone (http://www.ustream.tv).
- ❑ Check and save in your phone the local news media, sheriff's office, and emergency management offices including their blogs and Twitter accounts to follow during a disaster. Also include national agencies like Red Cross on Twitter at #howihelp.
- ❑ See Clark Regional Emergency Services Agency blog (http://cresa911.blogspot.com) for an example of a valuable blog before, during, and after an emergency.

Using Communications During a Disaster
- ✓ Use your personalized Google map on your phone or computer to locate household or family members.
- ✓ Use Twitter to reach household or family members who are separated.
- ✓ Use Facebook to post your whereabouts privately to your household members.

Communications in a Disaster 271

- ✓ Use your Emergency radio phone app to track news updates.
- ✓ Check news for real-time reporting on events (http://www.ustream.tv).
- ✓ Access your saved blogs, Twitter feeds, or news feeds for instant access in an emergency. Be aware that news on shelter and food is sent by relief agencies over social media sites, blogs, and news feeds.
- ✓ Use your saved Twitter hashtags to follow local breaking news.

Using Communications After a Disaster

- ❏ Update your location and status with your out-of-area contact person and others on your social media sites.
- ❏ Check the Google Crisis response site for up-to-date reporting.
- ❏ Use your phone apps to check your own vital statistics and data retrieval.
- ❏ Tune into YouTube and UStream for live feeds on disaster coverage.

In Summary

All regions of the world are subject to nature's powerhouse forces, while man-made disasters continue to dramatically impact lives everywhere. Out of the devastation vital lessons have been learned, resolve has been strengthened, and individual survivors and communities have risen to overcome their enormous challenges one day at a time. We now have more information than ever before to protect ourselves and our loved ones—even strangers—in the midst of a disaster. We hope that all will heed the wake-up call and will learn preparedness and self-reliance before any disaster occurs.

Throughout this book, we've shared how to prepare for natural and man-made disasters, outlining basic organizational steps to take in creating emergency kits, making a comprehensive plan, and developing broad and situational awareness. We have shown you how to reach out to your neighborhood, community, and larger area for information, training, and support. Checklists have been provided for food, water, and supplies to store, as well as how to build first aid kits. We have also reviewed insurance questions, safekeeping of important papers, interior and exterior hazards, and retrofitting. Before, during, and after sections for each disaster include lists of actions to take whether sheltering in place or evacuating.

Our resource guide offers timely details on smart phone applications and social media communications useful in any emergency. Chapters on each natural disaster, from seasonal thunderstorms, hurricanes, and tornados to earthquakes, landslides, and volcanic eruptions are provided with descriptions, explanations, and examples. Man-made occurrences, from chemical spills to electrical power outages, are also covered.

It is our hope that you are inspired to become more prepared and resilient in the event of any disaster. Refer back to this book often and feel free to reach out to us online (www.naturaldisastersbook.com) with questions, feedback, and comments.

Resource Guide for SmartPhone/Droid/iPad/iPod/iTunes

Below is an A–Z listing of the best of over 200,000 phone applications available, some of which you can add to your mobile device to prepare for a disaster. We have either tried these applications ourselves or have chosen them based on the highest and best user reviews. There is no shortage of phone apps, so let us know what you think, and be sure to visit us online (www.naturaldisastersbook.com).

Army Survival (Double Dog Studios) $1.99
- Over 1,400 pages and basic survival, evasion, first aid, and recovery information for staying alive in any environment.
- Requirements: Compatible with iPhone, iPod touch, and iPad.
- Requires iOS 3.0 or later

Bomb Threat Stand-Off (Applied Research Associates) $3.99
- Displays mandatory evacuation distances for eight different bomb types.
- Requirements: Compatible with iPhone, iPod touch, and iPad.
- Requires iOS 3.0 or later

Bump (Bump Technologies LLC) Free
- Cross platform sharing of texts, Tweets, Facebook, LinkedIn, shared locations, and contacts, etc. In the following languages: English, Chinese, French, German, Italian, Japanese, Korean, and Spanish.
- Requirements: Compatible with iPhone, iPod touch, and iPad.
- Requires iOS 3.0 or later

DocGPS (United Health Group) Free
- Locates the nearest doctor, clinic, or hospital anywhere in the world.
- Requirements: Compatible with iPhone, iPod touch, and iPad.
- Requires iOS 3.0 or later

Disaster Alert (Pacific Disaster Center) Free
- Interactive real-time hazards mapping all over the world.
- Requirements: Compatible with iPhone, iPod touch, and iPad.
- Requires iOS 3.1 or later

Emergency First Aid & Treatment Guide (phoneflips) $.99
- Printed hardcopy version sold over five million copies.
- Requirements: Compatible with iPhone, iPod touch, and iPad.
- Requires iOS 3.0 or later

Emergency Info (Blackberry) $ 2.99
- Emergency Info stores important personal information including your emergency contacts, current medical conditions, and past surgical procedures.
- Requirements: Device Software 4.2.1 or higher

Emergency Radio (Edgerift, Inc.) Free
- Emergency Radio tunes into live police, fire, EMS, railroad, air traffic, NOAA weather, Coast Guard, and other emergency frequencies.
- Requirements: Compatible with iPhone, iPod touch, and iPad.
- Requires iOS 3.1.2 or later

Flashlight (John Haney) Free
- Highly popular app turns your phone into a flashlight.

- Requirements: Compatible with iPhone, iPod touch, and iPad.
- Requires iOS 3.1 or later

HAZMAT Evac (Applied research Associates) $5.99
- Displays safe zones in a disaster taking into account weather and wind conditions for a chemical spill.
- Requirements: Compatible with iPhone, iPod touch, and iPad.
- Requires iOS 3.1 or later

ICE—In Case of Emergency (EMS Options LLC) Free (Blackberry)
- Provides EMT'S with critical personal and medical data: your name, who to contact, important notification telephone numbers, blood type, allergies, etc.
- Requirements: 4.2.1 Device Software

ICE4Family (EMS Options, LLC) $4.99
- Puts your family information together in case of emergency, and transfers information between devices.
- Requirements: Compatible with iPhone, iPod touch, and iPad.
- Requires iOS 3.1.2 or later

iCurfew (Infinity Curve© Radical Parenting) Free
- Uses GPS mapping to locate users of this app who can then send an untraceable email to verify location.
- Requirements: Compatible with iPhone, iPod touch, and iPad.
- Requires iOS 3.0 or later

Instant Heart Rate (Modula d.o.o.) $.99
- Measures your heart rate, and is available in two languages: English and German.
- Requirements: Compatible with iPhone 3GS,

iPhone 4, iPod touch (4th generation), iPad 2 Wi-Fi, and iPad 2 Wi-Fi + 3G.
- Requires iOS 4.0 or later

Line2 (Toktumi, Inc) Free
- Adds a second phone line to your device.
- Requirements: Compatible with iPhone, iPod touch (2nd generation), iPod touch (3rd generation), iPod touch (4th generation), and iPad.
- Requires iOS 3.1.2 or later

LogMeIn Ignition (LogMeIn, Inc.) $29.99
- "Leave your laptop behind" app in multiple languages: English, Chinese, Dutch, French, German, Hungarian, Italian, Japanese, Korean, Portuguese, Russian, and Spanish.
- Requirements: Compatible with iPhone, iPod touch, and iPad.
- Requires iOS 3.0 or later

Medscape Mobile (WebMD) Free
- The number one downloaded medical app in 2010 used by medical professionals.
- Requirements: Compatible with iPhone, iPod touch, and iPad.
- Requires iOS 3.0 or later

Paw Card: Pet Tracker for Your Dog and Cat (Jive Media LLC) Free
- Keeps your pets' vital information on your device.
- Requirements: Compatible with iPhone, iPod touch, and iPad.
- Requires iOS 3.0 or later

Pill Identifier Lit (Drugs.com) $.99
- Searchable database of over 10,000 pills for identification purposes.

- Requirements: Compatible with iPhone, iPod touch, and iPad.
- Requires iOS 3.0 or later

Orbit Social Phone Book (Trilibis Mobile) Free
- Mixes contact info with text, email, voice, and social sites; Facebook and Twitter, along with free outbound text messaging.
- Requirements: Compatible with iPhone, iPod touch, and iPad. Coming to Blackberry soon.
- Requires iOS 4.0 or later

POM Alert (ThinAir Wireless) $0.99
- POM (Peace of Mind) Alerts are location-based alerts with real-time notification, push notification, and GPS capabilities.
- Requirements: Compatible with iPhone, iPod touch, and iPad.
- Requires iOS 3.0 or later

Quake Alert (AppBanc, LLC) $1.99
- Alerts sent to your phone based on magnitude and distance regarding worldwide earthquakes.
- Requirements: Compatible with iPhone, iPod touch, and iPad.
- Requires iOS 3.0 or later

SAS Survival Guide (Trellisys.net) $6.99
- The very popular soldier scribed 20-year-old survival book on a phone app.
- Requirements: Compatible with iPhone, iPod touch, and iPad.
- Requires iOS 3.0 or later

Shop Savvy (Big in Japan Inc.) Free
- Turns any Google Android or Apple iPhone into a barcode scanner for finding the best deals from

local and online retailers. Use it when shopping for emergency supplies. This is the market leader.
- Requirements: Compatible with iPhone, iPod touch, iPad, and Android.
- Requires iOS 4.0 or later

Skype (Skype Software by S.A.R.L.) Free
- Video calling from your device in whatever language you need: English, Chinese, Danish, Dutch, Finnish, French, German, Italian, Japanese, Korean, Norwegian, Polish, Portuguese, Russian, Spanish, and Swedish.
- Requirements: Compatible with iPhone, iPod touch, and iPad.
- Requires iOS 3.0 or later

Smart-ICE (EMS Options, LLC) $1.99
- Smart-ICE and Smart-ICE4family, which stores data for up to eight profiles.
- Requirements: Compatible with iPhone, iPod touch and iPad.
- Requires iOS 3.0 or later

SugarSync (SugarSync) Free
- Synch files across multiple devices and access stored files. Available in English, Japanese, and Korean.
- Requirements: Compatible with iPhone, iPod touch, and iPad.
- Requires iOS 3.0 or later

Text Me! (TextMe, Inc.) Free
- SMS, IM, Photo, and Video Messenger in multiple languages: English, Arabic, French, Hebrew, Italian, Korean, Portuguese, Slovak, and Spanish.
- Requirements: Compatible with iPhone, iPod touch, and iPad.
- Requires iOS 4.0 or later

Twitterific for Twitter (The Iconfactory) Free
- A Universal Twitter app for your device to make sending and getting messages easier.
- Requirements: Compatible with iPhone, iPod touch, and iPad.
- Requires iOS 4.0 or later

Waze: Community GPS Navigation (Waze) Free
- It takes social driving to a new level. Users report speed traps and traffic delays in real-time.
- Requirements: Compatible with iPhone, iPod touch, iPad, and Android 1.5 and up.
- Requires iOS 3.0 or later

Weather HD (vimov, LLC) $.99
- The number one weather app in multiple languages: English, French, German, Italian, Russian, and Spanish.
- Requirements: Compatible with iPhone, iPod touch, and iPad.
- Requires iOS 3.2 or later

WebMD Mobile (WebMD) Free
- WebMD Mobile can check your symptoms, access drug and treatment information, and provide first aid essentials.
- Requirements: Compatible with iPhone, iPod touch, and iPad.
- Requires iOS 3.0 or later

X1 Mobile Search (X1 Technologies) $9.99
- "Leave your laptop behind" app in multiple languages: English, German, Romanian, Russian, and Spanish.
- Requirements: Compatible with iPhone, iPod touch, and iPad.
- Requires iOS 3.0 or later

YureKure (RC Solution Co.) Free
- Japanese language app for earthquake notification.
- Requirements: Compatible with iPhone, iPod touch, and iPad.
- Requires iOS 3.0 or later

Resource Guide— Recommended Websites

Amateur Radio Emergency Services
http://ares.org/

ASPCA—American Society for Prevention of Cruelty to Animals
http://www.aspca.org/pet-care/disaster-preparedness

FEMA—Federal Emergency Management Agency
www.fema.gov

FEMA—Spanish language site for preparedness and disaster assistance
www.listo.gov

Foursquare—Location-based social mobile platform
https://foursquare.com

Department of Homeland Security
www.dhs.gov

Google Crisis Response
http://www.google.com/crisisresponse/

Government site for before crisis preparation
www.ready.gov

Really Ready—non-government site that improves upon Ready.gov
www.reallyready.org

National Oceanic and Atmospheric Administration
www.noaa.gov

Tsunami information
www.tsunami.noaa.gov

Government site—access to disaster help and resources
http://www.disasterassistance.gov/daip_en.portal

National Interagency Fire Center
www.nifc.gov

Next Of Kin Registry (NOKR)
http://www.nokr.org

The Center for Disease Control and Prevention
www.cdc.gov

United States Search and Rescue Task Force
www.ussartf.org

Send Word Now—emergency notification system
http://www.sendwordnow.com/

Sahana Software Foundation—worldwide disaster
   management information
http://sahanafoundation.org/

Entity of the Department of Homeland Security's Federal
   Emergency Management Agency
www.usfa.dhs.gov

Resource Guide—Recommended Websites

National Earth Sciences Teacher Association
www.windows2universe.org

Science topics, NASA image maps, etc.
www.geology.com

American Red Cross
www.redcross.org

Know Your Stuff—Search for home inventory lists, insurance information, etc.
www.knowyourstuff.org

Emergency Preparedness Kits and Supplies
www.Homelandpreparedness.com
www.quakekare.com

National Flood Insurance Program
www.floodsmart.com

Emergency Foods and Kits
www.Nitro-pak.com

Earthquake preparedness company for Southern California
www.Earthquakecountry.com

U.S. Geological Survey
www.USGS.gov

The National Center for Missing & Exploited Children
www.missingkids.com

Hootsuite—Social media dashboard
http://hootsuite.com

Help displaced children from earthquakes
www.savethechildren.org

International Red Cross site to bring families together separated by disasters
www.familylinks.icrc.org

The Davidson Yell and Tell Foundation—Teaches children how to be a hero and take action
www.yellandtell.com

The Home Safety Council
www.homesafetycouncil.org

Private Homeland Security blog
www.nationalterroralert.com

National Fire Protection Association
www.nfpa.org

Site of March 1979 nuclear accident
www.threemileisland.org

Tweetdeck—Your social world
http://www.tweetdeck.com/

Ushahidi—Crowdsourcing/Mapping
http://www.ushahidi.com/

Internet TV
http://www.ustream.tv/

World Nuclear Association
www.world-nuclear.org

Article on the Minot Chemical spill
www.slate.com/id/2157395

Public site to help rebuild Joplin, MO.
http://rebuildjoplin.org/